DANCING
THE
RAINBOW

Lani O'Hanlon

Dancing the Rainbow

Holistic Well-Being through Movement

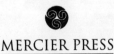

MERCIER PRESS

WHAT YOU NEED TO READ

MERCIER PRESS
Douglas Village, Cork

Trade enquiries to CMD Distribution
55A Spruce Avenue, Stillorgan Industrial Park, Blackrock, County Dublin

Sections of this book were originally published in
Network Magazine, Ennis, Co. Clare, 2000
For more information see www.dancingtherainbow.net
info@dancingtherainbow.net

ISBN 978 1 85635 546 9

10 9 8 7 6 5 4 3 2 1

A CIP record for this title is available from the British Library

Mercier Press receives financial assistance from the
Arts Council/An Chomhairle Ealaíon

Typeset by Dominic Carroll, Co. Cork
Illustrations by Fiona Aryan

Printed by CPI Mackays of Chatham. Chatham, Kent

To Laurie – thank you for the gift of dance

Contents

The Dance

Our aim in *Dancing the Rainbow* is not to be beautiful or expert but truthful in our expression of ourselves through movement and voice. We allow the body to move from the inside out, leaning into fears and disabilities, stiffness and rigidity, into the bones, joints, flesh, muscles, sinews and fluids of the body. We explore our physical body as a map.

The body expressing itself truthfully is the living sculpture of all that has shaped us.

The dance becomes a living art as we express our soul through the movements we make.

Our thoughts are still and our movements are the movements of birds and animals and winter trees. In this way we recognise each other and in the moment, we are free.

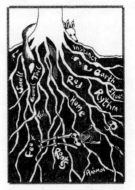

Introduction

Welcome to the Dancing the Rainbow, Movement, Sound and Colour Therapy Practice, a programme that works primarily with your physical body and then the more subtle energy bodies.

In *Dancing the Rainbow* courses everybody is welcomed. Communication takes place through our body language and tone of voice, and it is essential that we listen to what our bodies are trying to say so we are not giving out mixed messages and confusing ourselves and the people we love.

Did you ever wonder why you cannot move as freely and spontaneously as you did when you were a child? The colour therapy practice will show you where you are blocked energetically and physically and give you tools to free up and clear your energy. You will learn how to ground in red, work with your emotions in orange, improve boundaries, personal power and self worth in yellow, open your heart to yourself and others in green and pink and then go on to discover the attributes and clues in the other colours.

You will also discover practical ways to work with the inner critic and begin to move through self-criticism and self-doubt. You will then experience relief from the habitual, circular and stressful thinking that has become the norm in our society today. If you use the movement practices consistently, you will experience a release and recovery from addiction and trauma in the body and an increase in the vitality, energy, youthfulness and beauty that is unique to your body. As you progress you will find ways to communicate creatively through your body and restore balance, presence, fluidity and ease to your body and mind.

As you follow the explorations in the book you will become more and more intimate with your intuitive and instinctual body so that you dress for yourself, eat what will truly nourish you, play, create and live in a more authentic way. It doesn't take a lot of time but sometimes it takes a miracle because behind all that control and image we often don't like ourselves very much and are often filled with self-doubt. When we move differently, we think and see differently. Step by step DTR helps you to live and create in an authentic and holistic way that is in tune with your own organic process.

The first part of the book will tell you how this work was conceived and will describe the different tools we are working with. Then there is the 'Rainbow Warm-up' which is an introduction to the movement, body and energy work and can be done simply and easily so that you become familiar with different movements, energies, sounds and colours. Then there is some in-depth writing on my experience of 'Dancing with the Instinctual Body' over many years and finally the 'Dance Workshops' which will take you on a journey deeper into the rainbow colours and your physical and creative process. You can do one exploration from each colour or spend a few months on one colour or form a support group and work together on one exploration at a time.

The Roots

When I was a baby, my mother used to wheel me down to her dance class in the local school, the Presentation in Cork, and I would sit in my pram and watch the children from low infants to sixth class sing and dance. At age three, under the coloured lights, I tiptoed onto the stage for the first time in the Christmas panto. As a green and rust fairy bird, I covered the babes in the wood with leaves. These babes were adults and, as I looked at them lying there, I felt something akin to pity. I was not aware of an audience, just these two, lost in the woods. I was not lost then, my soul knew what I loved; the smell of tulle and make-up, the slippery sound of my ballet shoes, the rhythm patterns when I tapped, the sparkle of coloured sequins and snow-white socks.

I travelled the country with my parents and could be left for hours playing with coloured. I watched my mother perform onstage, teach dance and choreograph shows in diverse settings. She worked wherever she could, with every sort of community and theatre group, and, within minutes of entering the hall, she would be doling out songs, parts and dances. My father was a storyteller from Wexford and he taught me how to try new things and how to make a game out of earning a living. He also introduced me to the mysteries of storytelling, books, music and acting. As children we saw the bare, dark halls and how they could be transformed into places of wonder. We tidied up afterwards, saw the magic fade and drove home late at night. However, as a child and young adult, it was when I danced and sang alone and unobserved that I felt safe enough to begin to express, through dance and voice, feelings and desires I did not understand or know how to name.

Many years later, as a young mother, my creative work with dance and writing began to lead me deeper into myself. At first I found it hard to sit alone and simply be there in front of the typewriter and allow the words to emerge. I became depressed, physically unwell and unable to dance. A new surge of creativity was pouring through me, but I did not have the ground to hold it and my body would not let me tell the story I needed to tell. To find that ground I had to travel back through time, back into my body and my own roots. At the time I didn't know what was happening; it is only now in retrospect that I can see the wisdom of the healing journey.

Bodywork with a gifted psychotherapist, healer and teacher brought me below my thoughts and fantasies and into my emotional and physical body. The movements brought me down into my bones, so that my bones could tell my story, then my muscles, then my guts and finally my voice. My gestalt psychotherapist helped me to look at the movements I was making in a new way, encouraging me to let the movements lead me rather than interpreting them with my thinking mind.

And of course my body, like an old traveller, returned home to what I knew: the dance. At that time I did not know where these dance steps were going. I found music that I needed and gave myself the time and privacy to be this lone dancer, learning the movements as they rose up from the deep, sensing body. I worked in this way, every day and often through the night for some years. I also wrote diary after diary documenting my own creative journey and what was taking place in my body and mind. This was the only way to let go of the suppressed feelings crowding through my body. These body memories seemed to be coming not just from this one lifetime but from an ancestral memory encoded in my body. When I danced and trembled, shook and worked through who I thought I was and through the old fears, traumas and energy blocks, I was left with sweetness and a dawning compassion for my infinitely surprising and beautiful body.

This initiation took place over many years, in a housing estate, where I learned to dance with darkness in the hallway, in the kitchen and in the mountains around me. I was led to the wisest teachers, often ordinary people living in ordinary places, who had the inborn gifts of true artists and healers, and who studied and worked, paying for courses and books to hone their craft and to work with the often unbearable pain being healed at that time in our bodies and in the Irish psyche.

In the 1990s I was writing short stories and facilitating writing groups in Tallaght. Some of my writing buddies told me about this exceptional yoga teacher and they spoke so lyrically about her that I went to take a class. That teacher was Antoinette. When she was a young single mother, Antoinette went to live in the west of Ireland. Before she went there, she told people that she was going to learn about the elements. She lived in a thatched cottage with no running water or electricity; she cooked on an open fire and washed the clothes in a nearby river. Her knowledge, devotion and connection with the elements are embodied and her way of teaching, creating and being is instinctive. As an experienced yoga teacher, she understands that knowledge of the chakras, or energy body, is a body skill, like cycling or dancing. She also has a lot of experience working through the recovery process in the twelve-step programmes. She brings ancient wisdom and knowledge directly into our lives by speaking in simple, womanly, down-to-earth ways and demonstrating what she is saying with her body.

One night when she gave me a lift home I told her about my experience of dancing from the inside out and how I would like to show others how to do this. Antoinette turned to me in delight, 'This is my dream you are talking about.' This was the beginning of a creative partnership that lasted many years. Antoinette and I had ways of drawing each other out and making the other one name something that was emerging through her body. There was a yearning to express our creative gifts but because of sensitivity and a tendency to be overwhelmed by performance, huge amounts of information or task-oriented trainings, we were unable to do this in the structures available to us at that time. Almost without realising it, we began to create a space where we could subtly explore our spirituality, creativity and the dark, hidden places in our own bodies. We used movement (dance/yoga), colour and sound as a spiritual and creative practice and eventually called this practice Dancing the Rainbow (DTR).

People who attend a course in DTR typically name the following benefits:

- Less anxiety in the body and mind
- A deeper understanding and relationship with their own body, inner self and others
- A release and recovery from pain, addiction and trauma in the body
- More calm and stillness in mind and body

· A more creative and sensual way of life
· An increase in vitality, energy, youthfulness and beauty that is unique to one's own body
· Balance, presence, fluidity and ease in the physical body.
· A stronger relationship with their own instinctive knowledge and intuition

We often think that we should have before-and-after photos because of the way people change physically. You can see it in their eyes, facial expression and their way of holding themselves and moving. But DTR is not a quick fix and we often go through pain as we release old suppressed trauma from the body. The in-depth movement practice has a meditative approach to breath, voice and body-work and ways of working with the saboteur within. As we move through habitual thought and body patterns and re-educate the body, we begin to release dynamic, spontaneous, creative work and increase our physical and energetic presence.

Our medium is the clay of the body which has been moulded and shaped by our lives. DTR is an embodied and practical system that you do not need to 'go away' and practise but can do every day; in your kitchen or out walking. By reading, dancing and applying the exercises in your everyday life, you will come to reknow your own body. Most people do not fully inhabit their bodies; they are thinking, fantasising or spacing out. The first task is to fully embody – here and now. It takes many people years before they can allow the body weight to drop into the legs and feet and make real contact with the earth. Many of us go through our lives without any real sense of what it is to be 'at home' in the body. If we are able to fully experience the joy of the present moment and be present to our loved ones, our tasks and the nature within and around us, then this is true freedom. When we dance we experience this beingness – on our own and with each other – and it streams into the rest of our lives. It is a life-changing process.

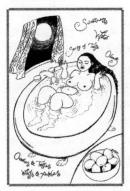

Colour, Movement and Sound

Clues/Attributes

Ancient spiritual teachings tell us that there are different attributes associated with the different energy wavelengths or chakras in the body. One night Antoinette was preparing for a class and she did a quick sketch of the body, filling in these attributes in a colourful, playful way. Her intention was to use them for that class. The results were so good that we began to use these clues/attributes and this little map all the time. I was studying colour therapy and I was very interested in the effects of colour and light on the movements we were making. After a while Antoinette and I began to see that these colours and attributes were clues to a body knowledge that was subtle and very powerful. We also discovered creative ways of playing with these clues, using them to inspire our dances, songs, stories, poetry and paintings.

I have always loved detective stories and it seems to me that each person has their own mystery and their own unique story, so dancing the different colours and exploring the clues is a way to explore that mystery. Each dancer begins to see where they are stuck or where they are sabotaging their lives, relationships and creative potential. They then have the knowledge and power to work with this, not as some strange or mystifying esoteric exercise but as a dynamic and grounded creative practice.

Put simply, we invoke the different clues we have learned

17

to use over many years; we do this visually through colour and image, sensually, by nourishing the body senses on every level and then through music, movement and sound. We then provide a safe and gentle environment where you can dance, sing and create without trying to live up to any standard or norm. As you explore the difference between the physical body, the emotional body, the mental body and the energetic body, you become clearer about what is happening in your own system, and you therefore become clearer in every aspect of your life. Communication is sharper; relationships are more intimate and authentic. You gain access to more and more creative potential in your life and work. Your body is able to release physical, mental and emotional trauma in a gentle, creative way. You begin to recognise when you are acting from distress, fear and undigested trauma and can begin to create new ways of being and acting. Your body then becomes freer and lighter as you are not pushing it and holding it in fear and distress but beginning the wonderful task of releasing your own body from the prison of your personal conditioning and the conditioning of the culture in which you live.

Healing and Creating with Colour

Colour, which is visible light, begins to melt the resistance, changes the vibration, softens and begins to heal the frozen trauma and chronic energy blocks in the body. Light helps us to move through the stiffness and fear without becoming bogged down by heavy, repetitive thinking.

When we begin to see with colour, our perception changes and we notice what colours we are working from and expressing and those we feel estranged from or uncomfortable with.

From the early civilisations to the present day, people researched and worked with the healing power of colour. The sun has been worshipped by many civilisations as they were aware that light and colour come from the sun. The Egyptians worshipped the sun and knew that without it there would be no light, warmth or life. They built temples of colour for healing where people could go to be revitalised and renewed.

Deep knowledge of the colours and their relationship with the chakra system and the elements – earth, water, fire and air – are used to inform daily life in most native cultures and this can be seen clearly in, for example, the cultures of the Navaho, Incas, Aztecs and Mayan and in our own Irish and druidic culture. The Judaeo-Christian tradition also refers to knowledge of the colours, for example in the story of Joseph with his coat of many colours. Knowledge of colour was once used to design the old churches and the vestments worn by the priests. In each culture there may be differences in how the colours and elements are perceived and linked, just as we have different languages, different food, different music and ways of dressing. However, each culture acknowledges the soul and the energy body in some way, and dance, song and art is an expression of this.

In Irish myths and lore, these energy centres in the body or in the land are often referred to as the seven gates. Myths are ways of going below the surface thoughts and finding the deeper underlying truth. The Irish myths speak of the veil being thin between the two worlds and the rainbow is seen as a mystical communication from the soul realms. The Irish language acknowledges daily the divine in nature: the elements are prayed to as we light the fire or listen to the wind, and the divine is acknowledged in every person we meet or to whom we bid farewell. The ancient Irish language is also poetic as is the language of the Aztecs and other ancient peoples; the poetic words are able to speak to deep layers within us. When speaking Irish, one is conscious of the vibratory power of words and the poetry of the soul. The language of colour and sound goes below words, but poetry, story, dream and myth intimates this energetic language and the language of the earthy, elemental forces moving through our bodies and our words.

The archetypal story of the Children of Lir is one that moves deeply in the psyche of the Irish, immediately connecting us with our mythical and spiritual past. We can also hear it in the prayers and blessings used in everyday conversation by our ancestors where the elements were honoured and prayed to every day:

> May the road rise up to meet you
> May the wind be always at your back
> May the sun shine warm upon your face
> May the rain fall softly on your fields
> Until we meet again, may God hold you in the
> hollow of God's hand (old Irish blessing)

The Inuit in Labrador say that sky dwellers live in the colours of the aurora borealis, the colourful lights that live on the crown of the earth in the polar regions of the north and can be seen during the long winter nights. The Inuit also say that they are spirits trying to communicate with the people of the earth and that some people have the power to call down the lights. These ethereal lights move in spirals and large veils of colour and it is said that the spirits are playing a game of ball; the players wearing lights on their heads and rainbow belts.

Myths, poetry, story, song, dance, prayers and artwork are the ways we have always endeavoured to give expression to the divine, to love, and the soul colours that breathe within and around us. Acknowledging the divine in the natural world can bring a sense of rhythm and purpose to the day. The mystic Rudolf Steiner, who had a deep understanding and knowledge of colour, nature intelligences and movement, created a movement practice called eurhythmy. He wrote and taught extensively and founded the Rudolf Steiner schools; he understood that many illnesses could be healed through the use of colour and he predicted that colour therapy would play an important role in the future. Schools based on his teachings use particular colours in the classrooms related to the developmental needs of the children. To go for lunch in our local Camphill café (places where people with special needs live in communities influenced by the teachings of Rudolf Steiner) is to feast the senses on every level. The paintings intimate the soulful life of the painter, the flowers and vegetables are coming in to us from the biodynamic garden outside where, through the window beside our table, we can see people with different levels of ability and disability working harmoniously together. The rugs there are woven with a sense of community and the natural dyes are easy on the eye. Woven baskets hang from the rafters and there are shelves and shelves of books to browse through as we listen to the music that has been carefully chosen. The books give us the theory, but it is the grounded, practical, spiritual practice that benefits everyone who comes through the door and the people who live, work and welcome us into their community. In this atmosphere we are nourished on every level. This is a very good example of the base chakra working well. In Dancing the Rainbow we endeavour to provide this community, if only for a short time. A beautiful place, food that has been grown and prepared with care, colours and images that soothe the soul and a safe space for people to move, dance and create together. In this way we can return to the ground of our being and gently heal developmental issues that relate to the different chakras.

Movement and the Chakras

Antoinette believes that balancing the chakras is the basis for many forms of energy healing: 'We can learn to tune our body instrument and let playful movement and expression of ourselves create harmony and healing in all dimensions of our lives.'

From the teachings of yoga, the Sanskrit word chakra means wheel or disc, and the chakra, when healthy, is a whirling vortex of energy. According to mystics and clairvoyants, these spinning vortices look like the petals of a flower, varying in number, vibratory frequency and colour. There are seven major chakras associated with the seven layers of the energy field or aura that surrounds the body. They are located at or near the body's major nerve plexus in the spine. There are twenty-one minor chakras. Each major chakra on the front of the body is paired with a counterpart on the back of the body. These chakras control the flow of energy into the body and between the various layers of the aura (the subtle energy bodies that surround the body) and the physical body. They also influence the organs and glands of the body. Each chakra is associated with a particular colour, sound, element and movement. A lot has been written in various books about the connection of the chakras to psychological and physical health. In Dancing the Rainbow we are using this knowledge as a creative/healing and spiritual path, but we do recommend and work with back-up support and help from the medical profession, psychologists/psychotherapists, complementary therapists and body workers of all kinds. Many enlightened healers from all disciplines are becoming more aware of these subtle energies so they can help people on every level.

The yogis went into deep meditation and many of the movements we use today came to them over time and through exploration and enquiry. Real yoga is a dedicated spiritual practice of mindfulness, movement and the development of compassion for the body and the body of the earth. The movement arises from stillness and sinks back into it. When we do movements that affect the different chakras and ways of being, we need to know what we are doing. Antoinette and I searched for relevant ways to teach and learn from this. Not just to teach it but to ask the question; is this true for me now, in my life today? What happens to me when I make this movement, when I am still, when I work with colour, when I tone? Can I feel these energies? Is the movement I am making affecting them? Is it bringing me stillness and wisdom not just in this class but in my life?

In other cultures, different words are used to describe these seven spinning vortices that are situated in different areas in the body. Because of the different frequencies and vibrations, these are usually seen as the seven colours of the rainbow. I would experience them as spirals of energy and strong physical sensations. This energy, which vibrates as different colours, emanates outwards into the energy field or aura like colours coming through stained glass. The energy mixes, moves, changes and blends together to form the aura (the colours/energy field around the body), similar to what we see in holy pictures where light emanates from the hands or surrounds the body of the enlightened being. The energy is more like air or even water; you can move through it and it can be changed like coloured smoke, with a thought, a vibration, a sound or a movement.

Although these seven major chakras or energy centres link the physical body to the more subtle energy bodies or aura, when we see with all the senses it is hard to distinguish the physical form from the light body. At times these seem to shiver together, as of course the physical body, although dense, is also made up of elements, energy and vibration. Ancient cultures knew this; our scientists are now rediscovering it, but when we try to explain everything in scientific terms it becomes disembodied, dry and lacking in full human intelligence. We need to dance it, sing it and let it inform our lives in creative ways.

Vibration, Music and Sound

Like emotions, energy or thoughts, the vibrations emanating through the body may not be seen physically but we can certainly sense and intuit them and they have a strong effect upon the body and mind. Some people can see the vibrating energy as colour, some can sense and almost smell and taste it and some people are polyphonic and can see music as colours and hear sound in the colours. The native peoples who live near the aurora borealis say that they can hear the sounds of the colours like a whistling and crackling. Most people are aware of the effect of music and sound and how it can resonate or vibrate deeply within us.

The healers of old knew the value of rhythm, vibration, sound and song. Hippocrates healed with sound. Pythagoras used music to soothe the minds of his disciples. Hazrat Inayat Khan, a musician who became a mystic and teacher, used his knowledge of rhythm and music to unveil deep and lasting truths. Ancient priests and healers used sacred geometry to produce harmonics.

The vibration and sound of sacred words have an effect on the whole system. Toning and chanting resonate through the body and influence wellbeing on every level. Drumming, chanting and dancing are used by every native tradition not just as entertainment or as a way to escape the pressures of life, but as a way of communing with inner soulful creativity.

In Dancing the Rainbow we have researched different music and sounds that resonate with the different colours and vibrations and the physical body. More and more we see a need to use music that grounds us in the physical body and resonates with the heart. As people seem to be driven more and more into their busy thoughts and beyond into cyberspace, there is often unacknowledged grief held in the heart chakra, and unconscious fear trapped in the organs, muscles, bones and cells. This causes deep levels of anxiety as the mind becomes more and more disconnected from the home of the body and earth.

Vibrations, colours and sounds are as much a part of the body as the nose or foot. The food we eat, the colours we surround ourselves with, the music and words we listen to, all of this has an effect on the vibrational body and our wellbeing. Although this writing requires that I try to *explain* what I mean when I use the word chakra or speak about vibrations, in DTR workshops we do not explain about energy or what the chakras are as a mental exercise, we demonstrate in the body and show people how to sense these different vibrations. Having shown the different movements and the energy and atmosphere associated with the different chakras / vibrations, people immediately recognise that they have already experienced these energies as thoughts, emotions and physical sensations but didn't know that these related to the different chakras. Having read about the work, you can discover this for yourself by dancing through the rainbow.

The Dancing Healer

From the beginning of time, bodies knew how to dance and they danced in order to commune with their souls. This is the work of the dancing healer – shamanic work that is known and recognised in most native traditions. Healers from cultures that were dismissed as barbaric or savage by the western world still hold the refined knowledge within their bodies.

In Ireland we still have our native healers who live close to nature and have cures passed onto them from generation to generation and there are a whole new breed of healers studying and learning and trying to understand the ways we need to heal our bodies, our minds and the earth. Music is still played and the healing effects of music are understood and respected. However, these ancient wisdoms are becoming swamped by addiction, materialism and greed.

Competition, suppressed trauma and stress eventually lead to addiction that eats into every area of our lives. In the dance, we are rediscovering and honouring the ancient roots of the dancing healer in our own bodies and racial memory, harmonising the knowledge with our lives today.

Movement / sound / colour, used correctly, move deeply into the body through the different senses. The combination of movement, colour and sound is very powerful and needs to be used carefully, otherwise the nervous system can become overwhelmed. For this reason, it is not something one can teach in a linear way. The work is cyclical and intuitive. I have witnessed profound and lasting healing through the intuitive use of these media. I have worked with groups and individual clients over many years, working through creative blocks, for example depression, frozen trauma and addiction, and I have been privileged to witness the effects on their lives and on my own. As we begin to unblock and recover, we are able to access our deeper creative roots and begin to give expression to them through movement in a simple and grounded way. In my experience this is best done when it is done gently and slowly.

You, the Reading Dancer

I have danced through these rainbow colours over and over for many years and each time I have discovered something that has helped me physically, emotionally, mentally and soulfully and, in turn, has helped my relationships, my creative work and the different people who danced with me over the years. We made many different discoveries as we danced the colours. Each person who dances with us has their own story and their own way of seeing and exploring; that is the beauty of the dance.

First of all there is the rainbow warm-up, which can be done any time, and any place. It can be done in five minutes or for much longer. Become familiar with it and you will understand it on deeper and deeper levels and you will be able to move through it with ease. In the dance workshops there are simple exercises, which I prefer to call explorations because I see us all as explorers – exploring uncharted territory, the sensing, vibrating body and the unknown landscape within. These explorations come from the bigger workshops and trainings and may seem deceptively easy, but they have come to us over time and are the result of extensive experience. It is what Antoinette and I have discarded that makes the work simple and effective. Go slowly, take your time; if you are going to use any of the explorations as a teacher or therapist, make sure you know them intimately in your own body first because we cannot teach what we do not know. This is an alchemist's journey and can only be discovered by the traveller, the wild dancer in you. There are no shortcuts. The surface mind may try to use the information to analyse inappropriately, but the alchemical knowledge contained in the body cannot be abused without consequences and one must approach the work with a good heart.

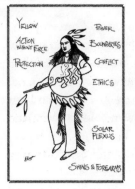

The Rainbow
Warm-up

This warm-up can be done in the morning or at any time to tune up the body instrument. Or you can use it as a warm-up before dancing any of the colours for a longer time. It can be done slowly or in five minutes before you leave for work. It is a way of giving yourself a daily dose of colour/light, meditation and movement and this nourishes you on so many levels.

By moving and oiling your joints and your whole body every day you are helping to prevent unnecessary wear and tear. By moving with awareness you can bring healing and health to your body without pushing, striving or forcing; you are not trying to achieve anything. If you are suffering with ill health or old injuries, move with care and do check with your medical practitioner. The movement in Dancing the Rainbow is intuitive and gentle. People of every age, ability and disability have danced with us. If your body hurts, you are not doing it correctly: stop, tune in and work gently, there is no force involved. If you find that you are getting irritated, angry or spacey, stop and breathe. Notice what part of your body you were moving. Were you trying too hard or pushing in some way? Slow it down, ground through your feet and hands. Be gentle, go more slowly. Even if you have very little movement available to you on any given day, sounding or breathing through the colours is healing and soothing on every level.

If you find that any of the creative explorations are overwhelming or triggering an old response in your body, then take responsibility and make a decision to stop. Say, 'I am stopping this now and may return to it later when I have taken care of myself in other ways.' Then seek appropriate therapeutic help if you need it. Be conscious about what you are doing; don't just abandon your body and your creative recovery. If you have any physical injury or difficulty doing the movements, then please consult with your medical practitioner.

The Body

- Before you dance, always warm and stretch your body first. Be aware that your joints, muscles, ligaments and tendons need to be warmed and stretched gently.
- See your spine and body as rigid plasticine that needs to be softened and made pliable. We use a small sketch through all the colours as the warm-up. It helps you to tune into and tune up each colour.
- Let your body move gently and intuitively; do not try to apply any remembered knowledge about dance, exercising or keeping fit. You are not trying to look beautiful; you are exploring your body knowledge. This gives you an instinctive and natural beauty that is all your own. Come from a beginner's mind; let go of the 'shoulds' and 'shouldn'ts' associated with how you look. Be childlike and simple. Sense into the mystery of your body using the colours as a map for your own nourishment and pleasure.
- Check out if my instructions are appropriate in your own body; if it feels wrong for you, then find some other way of doing it. If you trust the intelligence in your body, it will show you how to become more lithe and supple and you will extend your movement range and vocabulary. You can become healthier, suppler, more graceful and at ease in your body, gradually and easily. This is true for your mind and your emotions as well as your body; by moving, you still your mind and become more grounded, present, aware and your colours shine more brightly.

Preparing the Space

· Make sure that the room you dance in has nothing sharp to damage your feet, and no low stools or objects that you might trip over.
· Use natural fragrance, essential oils or fresh incense and you can light a candle and place it somewhere safe.
· If you are outside, put a flower or some other symbol in front of your body as a focus on the earth.

Dancing in the Different Colours

Each of these colours is associated with different physical and psychological states. As you begin to move through the rainbow body, you will discover where you feel balanced and in tune and where you are unbalanced and out of kilter. For example:

· The colour *red* and the movements in the base chakra are to help you come out of your head and habitual circular thinking and down into your body. If you feel anxious, caught up in your thoughts or spacing out of your body, then the movements here will help you to feel safer and more at home in your own body. They will help you to release old, stuck energy and trauma in the physical body. Moving here secures the ground to build on with the other colours and also helps to ground your dreams and creative projects. The movements here will connect you with your instinct, sense of smell, your natural rhythm, the skeletal and muscular system and support the whole structure of your body. If you have high or low blood pressure or heart problems, then substitute the colour green and turquoise.
· The colour *orange* and the movements in the second chakra connect with your sensuality, emotions, creativity, female power and taste for life. They will help you clear out old emotions, and past relationships that may be clogging up your system. By dancing here you become clearer emotionally and in your relationships. If you are feeling

dry, overworked and in need of a holiday, then even a few minutes connecting with this fluid energy will refresh and revitalise and give you access to a sweet, joyous sensation and the deep rest that comes from these reflective movements. These movements will connect you with the fluids of the body, encouraging lymphatic drainage and a healthy reproductive system.

· The colour *yellow* and the movements in the third chakra will help you to establish healthy boundaries and support the warrior energy we all need to deal with the world on a daily basis. The movements connect you to a sense of personal power, good boundaries, clear thinking, authority, assertiveness and autonomy, also playfulness and sense of fun. You will become aware of any self-worth issues so that they can be healed. If you are newly recovering from an addiction or burn-out, then replace yellow with the colour pink and calm the area by gently rubbing down the solar plexus area. The movements here will help you to focus, assimilate and eliminate on every level, including the digestive system. The colour yellow is also used to improve the eyesight.

· The colour *green* and the movements in the fourth chakra will connect you with your heart, breath, gentleness, gratefulness, simplicity, rest, ease, time and space. The movements awaken a sense of rhythm, balance, timing, simplicity and the ability to tune into your true desires and impulses with a childlike sense of awe and wonder. You will also begin to release old heart injuries that may be blocking you from a full, heartfelt connection with your life, other people and community. However, if you are grieving a recent bereavement then use the colour pink. The movements here will help with taking in, holding on and letting go. Green helps the cardiovascular system, inhalation and exhalation and the whole respiratory system. These movements also help to bring about a sense of balance in the body and in life, highlighting what to cherish and hold onto and how to let go so you are not trying to control events and other people inappropriately. You may also become aware of what and who nourishes you and where your energy is drained.

· The colour *blue* and the movements in the fifth chakra will connect you with your voice, your inner truth and creative expression in whatever form you enjoy; painting, poetry, gardening, singing and so on. You may also find that it evokes other soulful impulses; the desire to communicate in a deeper way or to listen to soulful music. It will also help you with public speaking, writing and with any blockage in the throat chakra or thyroid imbalance. If you have a fear of speaking or creating and suffer with a thyroid imbalance, use blue with green or turquoise. Sounding – using your voice and humming or toning through all the chakras – can heal on so many levels and brings more awareness and balance when speaking and listening.

· The colour *indigo* and the movements in the sixth chakra will connect you with your intuition, and imagination. Taking even a few minutes to dance and move here enables your inner visions and dreams to become clearer, more real and achievable and unconscious fears that may be holding you back will begin to emerge. If you are well grounded, then any psychic seeing will happen in a natural, easy way. If you have had negative experiences, nightmares or psychotic episodes, then replace the colour indigo with turquoise and work on the lower chakras with more emphasis, simply calming and balancing the upper chakras with gentle hands. The colour indigo can help ease pain and also affects the eyesight and the skeletal system.

· The colour *violet* and the movements in the seventh chakra will connect you with your higher creative inspiration and a sense of stillness and compassion. The light coming in through the crown chakra helps to alleviate depression or a sense of heaviness. If you are wearing violet or drawn to the higher movements, then it is essential that you have access to your creativity on a daily basis or you will become depressed and overwhelmed by the colour and inspiration that you are unable to ground. The colours and movements here can clear out the body and mind on every level, so use sparingly.

· *Magenta* and *green* help to polarise, balance and stabilise the whole system, especially after a shock or trauma of any kind. Use them after dancing through the colours and always end the rainbow warm-up by coming back into the base chakra so that you are grounded and balanced. Magenta also helps you with organisation and teaching and is a colour used by spiritual teachers with green to help them stay connected to the heart.

If you are feeling emotionally, physically or mentally over-whelmed, then substitute the colours pink and coral for the first four chakras and turquoise for the higher chakras (chakras 5–7).

By dancing through all the colours, you are listening to your-self on every level and also finding new ways of seeing and being. For example, if you are a very creative person but have difficulty promoting your work, the movements in sunny yellow and the third chakra will help you to project your energy and shine out-wards. If you are always out there with other people but feeling a bit burnt out and unable to access a deeper sense of yourself, then the movements in the orange and second chakra will bring you down into a more sensual, slower energy. If you are unable to access dreams or intuition, then indigo and the movements in the sixth chakra will bring you there. If you are suffering with writer's block or an inability to speak up for yourself, then blue/turquoise and the movements in the fifth chakra will help to balance the thyroid and give you the impetus to create and com-municate. Of course you need to go gently as you are entering a whole world of possibilities and I have written extensively on each of these colours (see 'The Dance Workshops', pp. 84–232). To begin with, it is important to heal and balance issues in the base chakra (the root), the physical structure of the body, as this provides the ground for the higher chakras to plug into. Without this base and structure, we are ungrounded and even though we may have great dreams and plans, we may not be able to realise them or we may find that we have to run too fast to keep up with our heads. The feedback I receive from people who are dancing the roots regularly is that they feel much less anxious and that they also experience a great sense of rhythm, ease and stillness within their own bodies. If you are finding it difficult to move because of physical injury or depression, simply find a place to relax, the floor or the bath, and breathe into the colours, visualising yourself doing the movements. Notice what muscles you would be using and what feelings come up in each of the colours. Keep it slow and safe. Play some gentle music that feels supportive and you can do a tiny dance with your little fingers. Even doing one small movement or dance with your fingers can be hugely effective, especially if you can do this in rhythm with your breath.

In colour therapy, the warmer colours complement the cooler colours and vice versa, so for a sense of balance it is important to be aware of this. For example, the complementary colour for the colour red is blue. If I am wearing a lot of red and doing a lot of base chakra movements, I may begin to feel rage or anger or simply overheated and hot and bothered. I can cool this down by breathing in the colour blue, wearing blue or turquoise and doing the blue movements. If, on the other hand, I am feeling blue and cold or spacey, I can use the earthier colours and the grounding movements to feel warmer and more connected to the earth. Once again, if you are feeling overwhelmed by emotions or circumstances, then do the movements but use the colours pink, coral and turquoise to calm and nourish your whole system. There are so many supportive therapists and medical practitioners of every kind, so there is no reason not to get help and support if you need it. However, you can do so much yourself simply by dancing through the colours.

So let's explore the rainbow warm-up with some simple movements:

- Begin by aligning your body instrument. Head and shoulders aligned with hips, and hips above feet, which are straight ahead and no more than hip width apart. Knees soft; ankles soft; hips soft.
- Stand still, let go, breathe, drop the body-weight into the hips and then down into the legs, knees, ankles, feet. Drop the shoulders, head and arms. Sink downwards. Notice sensations in your body, your breath, your heartbeat. Become still.

RED (Chakra 1): to come away from habitual thinking and worrying and ground into your natural, physical presence, power and instinctual knowledge.

Begin by noticing the physical sensations in the landscape of your body. Notice any aches or pains and also where there is a sense of wellbeing in the physical body.

- Notice where you are holding your body unnecessarily. Are your shoulders up towards your ears? Are you holding your neck rigidly? How about the base of the spine, your knees and so on? Notice your breathing. Is it shallow? Do not change anything, simply scan the body with awareness. Let the in breath touch these areas and let go on the out breath.
- Become aware of the base of the spine and give a little wag of your tail; feel that movement come right up through your spine.
- Let your heavy head sink down onto your chest and feel that stretch move right down the neck and spine into the base of the spine, the root. Breathe and let your head drop down more with each breath then gradually draw your head up onto the top of your spine. Open and close your jaw and feel that movement extend down through the spine and connect with the tail.
- Bring your awareness into your hands and feet. Bend your knees slightly. Hold your hands, palms downwards, so that

the energetic roots are extending from your hands and feet into the earth. Wiggle your toes and fingers.

- Push gently into one foot at a time: firstly into the ball of the right foot, then into the left. Then push into the heel, followed by the side of the foot. You are endeavouring to connect the sole of the foot with the ground by pushing gently into the ground.
- Notice the joints of the ankles, the knees and hips. Push downwards and release these joints one by one by pushing, holding, then releasing slowly.
- Move the different parts of your skeleton, leading with the joints. For example, move your arm, leading from the wrist, then the elbow, then the shoulder joint.
- Tune into your sense of smell; be aware of a connection between the nose and the tail. Wiggle your nose and your tail, you are connecting with the instinctual animal body – and the element earth.
- You can go on all fours like a cat, pushing the palms of your hands into the ground. Gently arch your back and then lower your back and raise your head. Do this a few times in rhythm with your breath. Then, when you are ready, come onto the soles of the feet one foot at a time, at first balancing your body by keeping your hands on the floor and then begin to push your self into a standing position, moving upwards one vertebra at a time from the base upwards, keeping the knees bent and soft
- Now, you can walk on tiptoe, then with your feet flat as you tap and stretch your feet. Stretch into your legs and buttocks and ease them out. Stick out your bottom, open your legs and wag your tail. Palms downwards, flat feet. Make low, groaning sounds from deep down. Open your jaws and show your teeth. The sound you can make is deep, low down, coming up from the roots: 'GRRRRR...'.

Red's complementary colour is blue.

ORANGE (Chakra 2): to sink into the female energy within, reflective, restful, intuitive knowing; sensuality and the emotional body; to enliven your juicy energy and taste for life.

· Notice what emotion is dominant for you today: Are you sad, fearful, happy or angry? Touch the emotion with your breath and surround it with a colour.

· Start by seeing a small thimble of orange fluid in the bowl of your pelvis and gently begin to swirl this liquid around by barely rotating your hips, first clockwise and then anti-clockwise.

· Increase the movement slowly and, when you are ready, begin to rotate your wrists one by one. Let your wrists lead, but be aware of the whole arm and the joints at the wrists, elbows and shoulders. Then find something to hold onto and rotate your ankle. Do this in a sensual way. Notice how all the muscles and joints are rotating right up to your hips. Lead with the knee, then with the big hip joint. Work evenly on both sides.

· Sense into the fluids of the body – your mouth, tongue and your sense of taste – by moving your tongue around the cave of your mouth and by licking your lips.

· Attune with the fluids in the body and visualise the colour orange juicing through the body.

· Stretch your hips. Push your weight into the right hip by bending the right knee and leaning towards the left side. Hold this position while breathing into any aches or tightness. Repeat on the other side. Ease out the hips by rotating and breathing into any remaining tight or stiff places.

· If you need to be awakened in this area, let the movements grow fuller, allowing the rhythm to come up from the base. If you need to calm the emotions in this area and if you are recovering from the recent break-up of a relationship or in the early stages of recovery from any recent trauma, then let the movements be gentle, more meditative (Hawaiian or Indian type movements) and visualise and breathe in

blue or use blue scarves, instead of the colour orange.
- Make sucking sounds with tongue and mouth and little groaning sounds deep down in your belly 'Mmmmsckmmtututusuckmmmmmmmmmmm'.

Orange's complementary colour is indigo.

YELLOW (Chakra 3): to connect with your active warrior energy within, ideas, good boundaries, self-worth, power, authority and autonomy.

- Notice what thoughts are dominant for you today and if your thoughts are speedy or slow. If they are speedy go easy here and use calming T'ai Chi-like movements. Watch the thoughts passing through your mind and let them disappear into a colour. If there are dominant thoughts or worries that keep cropping up, surround them with a colour. Breathe into the belly and the solar plexus and let out your fiery breath. Feel this whole area open up with your breath. Let out a 'haaa' sound.

- Stand firmly on the ground with your knees soft. Bring up your hand to shoulder level and slowly move your hand around to the back of your body, following the movement with your eyes. Go as far as you can and come back gently, lowering your hand. Now do the same on the other side.
- Move your hands and arms around your body, palms outwards, checking your boundaries and the space around you. Be aware of this boundary later in the day when you are with other people.
- Swing your arms around your body and, if it feels comfortable, throw out your arms in a loose rag-doll way. (Be careful not to have any objects nearby that you might hurt your arms on.)
- Move your shins and forearms by marching in time with your breath.

- Be aware of your eyes and gently focus them on a spot on the wall and begin to march towards that spot. Then turn sharply to the right or left, find another spot and march towards that. Your pathways through the room are straight. If you have a goal or an affirmation, you can bring that in here.
- Tune into the warmth in the body, the sunny yellow and the digestive juices by massaging the solar plexus area.
- The warrior movements are straight and karate-like, some-times sharp and sometimes sustained. Knees are bent and you drop the weight down into the legs and hips. Movements extend from the solar plexus. If you feel balanced and well grounded in the base, kick out your legs from the shins and your forearms – kung-fu style. Notice if you are pulling back into the shoulders and hips. Loosen these joints and let the movements be loose and easy. Make sure there are no objects that you might hit your arms and legs against.
- If you need to enliven this area, then marching is good. Eyes right – march right; eyes left – march left. Also good are charleston, tap, jive, hip-hop, rave and native warrior dances. If you need to calm and relax this area, Try T'ai-Chi-like or more meditative movements, but go gently at first. You may find it better to work with the first and second chakras for longer.
- To enliven this area, make sharp exhalation sounds, pull-ing in the solar plexus. 'Ha! Ho! Hee!' If you are feeling nervous or agitated, let the sounds be long and smooth 'Haaaaaaaaa–Hoooooooo'. Stay grounded in the base.

Yellow's complementary colour is violet. (These two colours together are very strong, so tone them down to gold and laven-der or mauve and pink if you need to.)

NB. If you are in the early stages of a recovery process from any kind of addictive pattern or substance addiction, then do not do the more fiery movements; work gently by rubbing and calming the whole area, making gentle sounds and then move on to the heart movements. You can add in boundary movements as you progress in your recovery and then gradually add in the other movements in the later stages.

GREEN (Chakra 4): to tune into your inner rhythms, breath, timing and self-love; harmonises and balances the whole system.

· Begin by moving one finger at a time, starting with the little fingers. You can close your eyes and feel the movement from the inside out. Be aware of all the muscles you are using just by moving your little fingers.
· Proceed slowly and move your other fingers slowly, then your hands, wrists, lower arms, elbows, upper arms, shoulder joints, chest and upper back, neck then head. Breathe and let the movements come from the breath with an awareness of your body moving the air around you.
· Move chest and upper back by breathing in and filling the lungs and opening the chest and arms and then breathe out slowly, rounding your upper back and pushing into the big muscles there; left side, then right.
· Open and close your arms, leading from the elbows. Rotate your shoulders slowly, forwards then backwards. Circle your knees and move your legs, leading from the knees. Dance around the room, leading with your elbows.
· Tune into the rhythm of your heartbeat, breath, your sense of touch, the colour green.
· Movements can be playful, skipping or opening your arms as if you were flying through the air.
· Open your heart to life; now cuddle your arms around your upper body. Give a big stretch, pushing your hands and arms upwards and standing on tiptoe, then slowly sink downwards, letting the arms and hands bring you down.
· Move your hands around the back of your body and in the space above, below, behind and around.
· You are looking for balance in the heart and simplicity, rest, time, space.

· If you are working with a lot of suppressed grief, then let your colours be soft pink and gold and the movements gentle but grounded.

· Make a connection to the roots by pushing into the feet and hands.

· Make a heart sound in the upper chest and back. Pat your upper back, shoulders and upper arms gently – Sound: 'Haaaaaaaaa', like you would say to a baby while patting his back. Magenta, which is a mix of violet and red, can be used with green to balance and polarise the body after a shock.

In colour therapy, green does not have a complementary colour as such.

BLUE (Chakra 5): to help you listen to the little whispers, your own truth and creativity; helps with performance, public speaking, writing, artwork, singing, acting and creative blocks.

· Open and close your mouth and make funny faces. Make small sounds, groans and moans. Massage your neck, let your head drop slowly downwards. You can curl right over, knees bent, head, shoulders, solar plexus, hips. Hang like a rag doll, then rise slowly, one vertebra at a time – hips, solar plexus, heart, shoulders – finally neck and head. Make sure there is no pressure on the spine or the knees.

· Move your upper arms and thighs. Wobble the flesh on your thighs, buttocks and upper arms. Tune into sound – LISTEN.

· Look upwards into the blue, use movements to draw down the cooler colours and the inspiration. Raise your arms in the air and pull it down.

· Open your mouth and close it like a fish. Make raspberry sounds with your lips. Then smacking sounds. Shake your head from side to side, wobbling your cheeks and lips and making wobbly sounds. Stick out your tongue and make sounds by moving it around your lips. 'Blah blah' gibberish.

Make funny faces and sounds. Do funny laughs. High pitched. Low down in the belly, tittery, high posh-lady laugh, deep, hearty, man laugh. If you have difficulty making sound, then start with gentle humming.

· Move your lips and let the sound come from different parts of the body floating upwards and downwards through the colours. Sound: 'Bluuuuuuuuuu . . . aaaaaaaa . . . eeeeee . . . oooooo'.

Red is the complementary colour for blue.

INDIGO (Chakra 6): to tune into your intuition, visions, dreams and destiny.

· Do a little trance dance by gently tapping your heels on the ground and making a little sound down low in the body. Attune with the colour indigo which is the colour of blue ink with purply undertones. Movements are American-Indian-like. Soft feet.
· Drop the weight downwards. Let your body and face be soft and relaxed. Eyes – soft focus.
· Make a little repetitive sound, 'Hey Hey – Hey Hey'. Move around the room and let your body be loose, a clackety skeleton bouncing on top of your heels. Your head is loose like a puppet.
· When this feels complete, gather the energy at the top of your head with your arms and hands, join your hands and put them on the top of your head, then in front of your forehead, then heart; now gently open your hands and send the energy down into the ground.
· Make a nasally sound in the nose and forehead, like a droning bee sound, or 'nee naw, neeng nong'.

Orange is the complementary colour for indigo.

VIOLET (Chakra 7): communing with the sacred, inspiration, meditation, stillness.

- Move the colours around your head. Let your hands linger at the top of your head, gently balancing the energy there; now move your hands around your body. Use ritual and sacred movements as you clear and clean the energy field in and around your body.
- Check that you are still grounded in the base and not floating off. You can make sounds and clear the energy in the room as you dance through the space.
- Sense the tingling in the tips of your fingers. See if you can feel that tingling right through your whole body. It can feel grainier in the lower chakras and finer around the heart. Notice the tingling on your face and around your mouth. Become still. Become aware of the energy dropping down through your body from the crown and coming back up from the earth.
- Let your face and jaw relax. Close your eyes, accept all feelings, sensations and thoughts by becoming fully present to them; let all cares and worries be held in the light.
- You can finish by gathering all the colours in the palms of your hands and feeding them into any of the places on your body that need tenderness and attention.
- Sound: High humming 'Mmmmmmmmmmmeeeeeeeeeeeee...'

Yellow/gold is the complementary colour for violet. These two colours together are very strong and need to be used sparingly.

Finally, notice where you still feel stiff or tense and move that part of your body. Let your body give a little shake. Ground the body in the red again. As you practise dancing in the different colours, you will grow more accomplished in this little warm-up. You can warm up through these wavelengths every day and you could do it in about five minutes. Or you can warm up before you dance one of the colours for a longer time. To polarise and balance the whole system, breathe in green horizontally through the heart.

Breathe in magenta (a fusion of violet and red), red in through the feet, and violet down through the crown. Use your hands to brush off any stuck or stagnant energy. Briskly stroke your body from the head downwards until you reach your feet. Squat down and place your hands on the earth; give thanks. Thank the colours and your body. Find your balance again. Become still. If you do not want to work with one of the colours, use a subtle version of it; for example, peach instead of orange or pink instead of red.

Short Version of Rainbow Warm-up

Red   Push your hands and feet into the earth and wag your tail. Do a little rhythm tapping of your feet on the earth. Breathe through your nose and smell the air. Wiggle toes and fingers.

Orange Circle hips, wrists and ankles. Move as if you are moving through water or as if you are water. Make sucking noises with your mouth.

Yellow March. Feel the yellow sun shining outwards from your solar plexus. Move your hand and eyes slowly from the middle of your body to the right then back to the middle and down. Repeat on the other side. Now march slowly.

Green Open and close your arms in rhythm with your breath. Touch your body firmly and gently.

Blue   Hum while swaying from side to side.

Indigo Smooth out your forehead and eyes with the tips of your fingers.

Violet Put your hands in the prayer position on the crown of your head, then forehead, then heart and then open your hands and extend them downwards, palms towards the floor.

Finish by breathing up magenta from the earth and down from the crown and breathe in green horizontally through the heart. With the palms of your hands, briskly brush your body from the head right down to the feet.

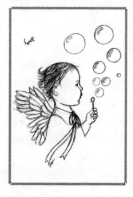

Dancing with the Instinctual Body

In our workshops and training we always begin with extensive work on the base chakra – the physical earthy self, the natural instinctual body – and this informs all our work in the other colours. As we work with the other colours we return again and again to the base chakra to ground us and to integrate the work in the other chakras. At the beginning of the workshop we first of all become still, to pause, listen and focus. In all our work we begin from the still point. We draw back our judgements from our own bodies and from the people around us. We all have habitual ways of looking at ourselves and other people and making little judgements based on our conditioning. By taking a moment to draw these habitual thoughts away from the body and from other people, we leave our bodies free to express themselves.

For example, if you meet people who knew you years ago when your were a certain way, and they still see you that way, you may find yourself reverting to that way of being even though you have outgrown it. In the same way, if we project our limited thoughts onto our bodies and the other bodies around us, we are constricting the energy in the bodies because we are sensitive creatures and we do pick up on other people's thoughts. When we do this simple clearing, we can literally feel the space in our circle clearing and the bodies relaxing now that the onslaught of constant thought and judgement has been turned down.

We also visualise or draw back all the energy we may be

projecting out onto other people, places and activities so that all of our energy is available and we can land, here and now. We then allow the body to reveal itself; this little pain here, that stiffness there, the longing for a big stretch – oohh just there – or a scratch – oh yes – just there. We give the body permission to express what it is feeling and sensing, let it move into different shapes, low down on the floor or stretching high, or curled up in a foetal position.

Dancing earth we use drums and rhythmic music and we have earthy colours on the light boxes and scarves and muslin and also the gentler blues and greens for balance. We dream into these colours and come up with volcanoes, and the fire at the centre of the earth. Or thick packed muck, soft squidgy muck, gentle clay, sandy desert, and sand being blown by the wind. We use our feet to explore this; for example, dancing in wet muck and finding ways of working with the imprint of our feet, walking on sand, using sand to play with or making sand sculptures or mud pies, taking photographs of painted feet or playing with our feet. We contact the element within our bodies and we explore earth walks. We might ask people who are earth signs to show us how they walk. We are beginning to play the game: earth.

Around the room we have grounding, earthy images, little altars with a theme we have been drawn to ourselves; for example, photographs of wild animals, bones, branches, a skeleton. We encourage you to stick out and shake your bottom, to bend your knees and explore rhythm by dancing your bones – clicky, clackety – as if you were a skeleton dancing round the room. You can lie on the ground or the earth and tap out rhythms with hands and feet. This helps you to explore rhythm and check into what your rhythm is like today. It could be slow and even or definite and fast or speedy and out of rhythm. The first rhythm was the rocking of our mother as she held us in her womb and the rocking of the little baby in the cot. To connect with this rhythm, our focus comes down to the feet and now we might like to check how we are balancing on the earth. Do you walk up on the balls of your feet, or do you dig your heels into the ground? Or perhaps you walk with more emphasis on the right foot? As you move or dance, you might acknowledge physical pains or aches and the way they influence how you move; for example, there is pain in my left shoulder; my right foot is turning slightly in or my feet are very stiff and my legs feel heavy; I have varicose veins; can I do anything about my falling arches, the ache in my lower back? I feel like jumping up in the air with exuberance, there is a huge amount of energy in my tail! At first people may not notice any of this. That does not matter; the body is leading and knows what to do.

Our first task was to grow. To develop the physical body, all of the parts linking together from the tiny sperm and egg to the cells, blood, bones, muscles and flesh; to embody on earth. Energetically, that body holds whatever truths and gifts we are bringing to earth and also old patterns and pains from our human, psychic past. The body we choose carries the ancestral line and country of origin with its tendencies, culture and past. It carries the inherited illnesses and emotional scars of our clan. Deeper again, it carries the god/goddess root, our sacred heritage, an ancient knowing of who we really are.

Just think of the fascination we have with a baby and the way it is going to grow. ('I think it takes after my side', 'No, the nose is just like his grandmother's'.) As the baby begins to grow physically, it will remind the parents of themselves and their respective families. It will know how welcome it is on the earth, and can tell how much it is loved. As it develops, its body shape will be moulded by all of this.

A Sense of Place

The land we are born in has shaped our parents and their parents; it has shaped our bodies and the way we speak, think and see. Our landscape tells the story of its people. In Ireland my history is written in the standing stones. My psychic past lies in the old stone shelters and houses; in the cairns and under the bog. Clues to our secrets lie hidden in the landscape.

Because of Irish roots of poverty and hardship, our inheritance of oppression, emigration, alcoholism, incest, religious abuse and mental illness, we may want to run from the past and the landscape around us. Affluence shows itself in the new houses that have appeared on the land but which have not grown out of her. Our ancestors used the local materials to build and, as I heal my past with its famine, pain and mystical memory, I begin to see the simplicity, craftsmanship and beauty of it: the whitewashed cottages on land that undulates to the sea; the red splash of wild berries and painted doors against the blue-grey mist; the swish of an island woman's red petticoat in the days before electricity. It is from her I came; she cut turf for the fire she cooked on and prayed over, her water came from dark moist earth.

Born from Irish earth, I carry her pain and her shame. I also carry her knowledge and creativity, her mystical and mythical past. The diddley-eye music we were once ashamed of and tried to hide is in my blood and bones and now I see it emerge from the wild places and stream around the world. All this and more becomes part of the dance as we find ways to dance our roots.

My mother ate boiled nettles from the garden. A relative on my father's side was a hedge schoolmaster who taught the children in the fields during penal times, when an Irish education and learning the language was forbidden. These are my roots and sometimes with the east wind they pull at my feet. This is my place, my dance: I can reject it or leave it. My tongue that always feels a little stiff when speaking or writing in English and the fear and confusion that comes when I try to remember school Irish; these are my roots, you have yours.

It is this clay we are given, to mould and shape. The landscape of the body, then, can teach us a lot. It holds the clues and creative seeds to who we are and why we are here.

The body is sacred. Although 'I' am not my body, my body tells a lot about who 'I' am. Wherever we live, if we want to set down roots, we need to go to the elders of the land or the ancient landscape and learn from them. Even if the people reject us, that too can inform our dances, our poems and our songs. Land that we resonate with never rejects us, and sometimes the stranger can see and love the land more than those who were bred there.

Grounding

You carry in the cells of your body a memory of everything that happens from the moment of conception right through birth and onwards. This is the ground you build on. When this has been damaged, the ground is shaky and you feel unsupported and afraid. Your roots are not able to support you. However, when you create from these roots and begin to express what that was like for the body, you can create a dance, a song, a painting, or simply make a sound and a shape. We are returning to that old ground in a safe and gentle way. When we acknowledge and accept our old wounds, we become more human and the body softens. Slowly we begin to make it safe in the here and now. Some of you may say, 'Oh, but I had a good childhood, my roots are good.' Thankfully there are children who have good and nourishing childhoods, but no child on earth escapes emotional and inherited pain. When you dance your roots, you may find that the healing is taking place not just for you but for your ancestral line and your relationship with the earth and the different peoples on earth. I have found that there is nearly always a sense of disconnection in the root chakra because the way we live now forces us to think too much. As young children we are forced to sit for long periods of time in seats and chairs that do not support the spine correctly, and this at a time when the physical body is growing and needs light and exercise. Instead we begin to develop the mental body too early and this replaces the natural puppy exuberance and the intimacy that comes when children roll around in the grass together or lie down to sleep together. Instead we are separated out in to solitary little mental worlds with the overuse of computers and televisions and the emphasis on academic achievement or competitive physical activity. Long periods of time are spent travelling in cars, bent over schoolwork or dazed by television. In his last letters, the artist Gauguin saw what this kind of education was doing:

> Soon the Marquesan natives will be incapable of climbing up coconut trees, incapable of going into the mountains to look for the wild bananas that can provide them with food. The children are kept in school, deprived of physical exercise, their bodies always clothed (for decency's sake); so they become frail, unable to spend the night in the mountains. They have all begun to wear shoes, and their feet, being sensitive from now on, will not be able to run along the rugged paths, or cross streams by stepping from stone to stone.
>
> So what we are witnessing is the sad sight of a race becoming extinct.

He also spoke about the innate artistry that could not be seen by the so-called educated missionaries:

> None of these people who claim to be so educated had any idea of the value of the Marquesan artists. There was not one official's wife who did not exclaim, on seeing examples of the art: 'But it's dreadful! It's just plain barbaric!' Barbaric! That's their favourite word. Any of the women can make her own dress, plait her hat, bedeck it with ribbons in a way that outdoes any milliner in Paris, and arrange bouquets with as much taste as on the Boulevard de la Madeleine. Their beautiful bodies, without any whalebone to deform them, move with sinuous grace under their lace and muslin chemises. From the sleeves emerge essentially aristocratic hands. Their feet, on the contrary, which are wide and sturdy, and wear no laced boots, offend us but only at first, for later it is the sight of laced boots that would offend us.

We can read this now and wonder at the ignorance of the missionaries but all of this is in our physical and mental make-up.

When I took off my shoes on the road because my feet were sore, my small children were embarrassed for me. When I asked some young people to remove their shoes for a dance class, one girl said that she hated feet. And many of them were embarrassed by their bare feet and wanted to wear socks. When I asked them how many experienced difficulty going to sleep at night because they couldn't stop thinking, they all raised their hands. When I am teaching dance in my bare feet I notice how people glance down and then away as if I had exposed myself. When I look at people's feet they often look dead and lifeless with very little movement available in the toes. They also look squashed and deformed from being in shoes that are made to fit a pointy foot. If we consider that these are our roots, then how can the plant above be healthy?

Rhythm

The person who has no rhythm physically cannot walk well; he often stumbles. The breath, the speech, the step all have rhythm. The person who has no rhythm in his emotions falls easily into a spell such as laughter, or crying, or anger or fear. We should practise rhythm in our lives.

Hazrat Inayat Khan, *The Mysticism of Sound and Music*

I am watching my daughter onstage; she is tap-dancing with other young men and women. Their teacher is gifted. She studied with tap masters in America, and in her choreography I can sense her rhythm and playfulness and also a fresh wave of spontaneous street-dancing that is low to the ground with its own roots in native dance. They are combining intricate tap rhythms that require great flexibility in the feet, ankles and knees, with African drum rhythms. To tap-dance well, you must trust the intelligence in your feet; to drum, you trust your hands. Onstage now, they are playing with rhythm, cleverly building layer upon layer. This is communicating to something within me that exults in the power of it and the lighthearted way they are dancing it.

My daughter is smiling, she knows she is playing with something below thought, the intelligence in rhythm that is quicker
than thought. If you stop to think, you lose the rhythm. This
is what the mystics mean when they speak about being fully
present. Not a spaced-out dreaminess, but a vital presence that
is now, now, now; alive, awake, the whole body vibrating energetically with this pulsating, life-giving rhythm.

In every culture down through the ages, from Spanish flamenco,
African drumming and dance, tango, salsa, clog-dancing, to traditional Irish dancing, a talented rhythm maker will bring us to
life. My daughter told me about her experience with this mixing
of rhythm and how it is impossible to think. 'If you think, you go
wrong.' She was laughing. 'Some other part of you has to do it.'

There must be no thinking, only that split second when your
sound comes in a fraction of a beat behind another's and each
person's sound is equally important: the ones holding the basic
rhythm and the fancy foot workers. The whole dance does not
last long enough. They build and they build it – then, *stop*!

The audience yells in delight. 'Do it again.'

It's over though, and I am glad I was paying attention while
it lasted.

Can I pay that attention to the rhythm of my life?

I am sitting in a hotel in Killarney. It is full of people attending a seminar. A young musician is walking out of the room
when an older one stops him. They both fish out tin whistles
and, regardless of the people around them, begin to share a tune.
The older man's hands on the whistle are tender, eyes laughing,
soft. The young man's body is as lean as the whistle, every muscle and bone playing the tune. In the middle, for no apparent
reason, he raises his foot and stamps it on the floor. It stomps
into a silent beat just behind the notes. With that stomp, I realise I could hear that silent beat. It is not just the music, they like
each other, there is recognition and an old connection. Their
body rhythms are longing for an expression of that attraction,
and they have the dexterity and musicianship to relate to each
other in a way that delights us all.

This is what brings people together to tap hands and feet and diddley-eye. We play spoons, and *bodhráns*; or clog-dance. These old rhythms call us to a wildness that brings us down, down to where rhythm lives.

A Kerry man called Pat was telling me about dancing in the houses years ago. One of the customs was that you did not show the soles of your feet, which kept you very low to the ground. The chief dancer stood on the flagstone in front of the fire. He was the focal point. Underneath the flag had been hollowed out and old skillet pots thrown in, creating a kind of vacuum, the sound of them banging in time to the chief dancer's feet. This sound gave him authority as he dictated the rhythm to the musicians and the rest of the group.

A good rhythm maker will use that authority wisely. A dancing healer will use it to heal the body, the mind and the soul.

Hazrat Inayat Khan tells us that in some cultures if a person yawns, another person claps. This is working with rhythm. A good musician or dancer will not even think about it. They know when to bring it up and when to slow it down. Hazrat Inayat Khan, a musician who used his knowledge of music to become a spiritual teacher, also wrote that he could tell if a man was out of rhythm when he walked in the door by the way he had fastened his tie. He also said that the entire mechanism of the body is working in rhythm; the beat of the pulse, heart, head, the circulation of the blood, hunger and thirst all show rhythm and the breaking of that rhythm is called disease:

> In ancient times, healers in the East, and especially those in India, when healing a patient of any complaint of a psychological character known either as an obsession or an effect of magic, excited the emotional nature of the patient by the emphatic rhythm of their drum and song, at the same time making the patient swing his head up and down in time to the music. This aroused his emotions and prompted him to tell the secret of his complaint, which hitherto had been hidden under the cover of fear, convention and forms of society.

The patient confessed everything to the healer under the spell produced by the rhythm, and the healer was enabled to discover the source of the malady.

We can also hear it in conversation. The person who is always just that bit off-key or coming in at the wrong time with the wrong word or laugh. Nervousness or shyness can throw us off, but some people are just off, depending on whom they are talking with or where they are. That could be another culture or in a different part of the country or with a group of people who do not accept them. Their rhythms just don't seem to match. Or someone telling a joke and the little silence from his audience is just that bit too long, his laugh a little off. In comedy, timing is everything.

Leading a group is all about going with the rhythm and pacing the work. Once again it's about weaving our rhythms. If I am working with a dancer, there are times when it's a good idea to bring us both out of the chairs and explore a little movement. There are times when it would be totally wrong. How do I know? I am tuning into their rhythm and another rhythm that is directing us from just behind our breath.

Often people seem to have trouble with rhythm, either holding it in dance or even drumming a simple rhythm. They find it hard not to speed it up or they go dead with it or just lose where it is supposed to come in. They can become impatient or angry or just lazily not bothered. If they can contain these feelings and gently stay with the process, these are the very people who become good rhythm makers.

When this happens, that person's whole body make-up changes. I see people who have all the energy up around the head and chest with thin torso and thinner legs. I see them approach other people with the head held awkwardly on top of the spine. A bit out of balance and coping with it, but something is out of sync in their lives and they know it. I can see when they get the rhythm that a new confidence starts to come into the body: a balance.

It feels like little electric currents that weren't working in the brain begin to connect from the right to left and left to right and from the feet up to the head. Particularly working with African rhythms or songs that are different to rhythms I learned before, my brain says, 'I can't do that, that's odd. I don't know how.'

Then after a while when Torsten Eisenberg, our drummer, is working with a call and response and simple clapping rhythms, I sense something zinging in my head and feet, and currents rippling through my body's systems. It pickles my old way of thinking and seeing.

After these rhythm, dance and voice sessions, life opens up and we can find new ways, new channels, jigsaw pieces that were always missing. Hand-eye co-ordination, inner timing and rhythm, all of these find new ways of communicating with each other. New internal pathways are created in the nervous system that release distress and cloudy, distressed thinking that comes from old developmental trauma.

Experiencing this new way of being is akin to being let out of prison. Working strongly with rhythm and voice in DTR, I was dreaming that I was trying to play a complicated piece on the piano without ever having had a lesson. In the same way, I remembered trying to do tap steps as a child before I was ready for them, and feeling frustrated and almost ill: a familiar feeling to me now and a gut warning that I am going out of rhythm, taking on too much, going out of step and out of tune. To teach something in a rhythmic and grounded way is to enhance the body knowledge and intelligence in other people, and to draw out their natural, rhythmic way of learning and recognising what they already know. This increases confidence and, even if we know one thing really well, one little rhythm step or simple drum beat, the fun and passion in us will play with it and draw it out and expand it; so we are in charge, with easy access to the playful child who loves to learn. The native teachers teach like this, telling the story over and over and adding something a little different each time. A good dance teacher will do the same.

Teach one step, and then when the student really knows it, only then do they show them the variation; they teach from the feet up and there is a great sense of joy and adventure.

Rap is popular, and it is easy to remember words and verses when they are set in a rap. The whole body is involved in a rap; the mouth, the tongue and rhythm coming up from the tail. Often the young singer who is rapping is telling us some heavy truths about their life. Street dancers and rappers are often fresh and spontaneous, more authentic than stylised bodies trying to produce overcomplicated steps, ideas, concepts, etc.

After these dreams, I discovered that I was writing, creating and playing in a passionate rhythmic way that was totally new for me but had echoes of familiarity. Saying to myself, 'I always knew I could do this, I just didn't know how.'

Also I was pacing myself, whereas before I would work non-stop, then collapse and give up. Can you recognise any of this in your own body?

When children with learning difficulties are given rhythm workshops, they heal in ways we cannot even imagine. However, the rhythms need to be simple. Unfortunately we can over-complicate things and always pile on too much for every learner; in schools and universities it seems to be a virtue to overwhelm people with information and criticism and then watch them struggle to cope. This creates the feeling of being a failure and fosters an inability to stick to something. It affects our commitment to life and learning, when we make it too hard or it is made too hard for us. People take in a certain amount intellectually, but it does not filter down into their lives, their relationships or the bones of their bodies and so they feel like they have to spoof it a bit because they know, deep down, that they don't really know.

I was teaching some children a dance and there was one little boy, Declan, who looked on disdainfully and declined to join in. Another boy, Luke, couldn't contain himself to learn the steps. He was so filled with exuberance that he had to jump around and I noticed that there was a lot of high energy up around his head. However, when he spotted the bongo drums he became really interested, bashing at them and waving his head around. 'That's not how you play the drums,' I tossed at him. 'That's noise; if you want to learn I will show you.' I went on teaching the others the dance and after a while he came and asked me how to play. I began to teach him a simple rhythm; because he was so interested, he contained the wild, exuberant energy and then gave vent to it on the drum. He kept trying to rush it. He really found it hard to hold the simple rhythm but eventually he started to get it and with a little praise he began to flush with pleasure. Then Declan, who had been looking on disdainfully, tried to grab the drum and even though he gave me a dirty look he agreed to learn the rhythm with another drum. Because they really wanted to learn, both of these boys were able to and they drummed along in time to the dancers. Luke has been diagnosed with an attention deficit disorder, but I felt that his sense of rhythm was a little out of kilter with the others and somehow he knew it. Instinctively he knew as well that the drum would help him give expression to his own rhythm and of course he would get to make a lot of noise! Declan was using his disdain as a defence. I think he was afraid of making a fool of himself by trying to dance but because Luke was so prepared to do it all wrong, this gave him the courage to try.

Learning is such a private, personal thing; we all learn differently and we don't necessarily learn well when we are made to stay sitting. Many new educators are discovering that people can learn almost anything if they are jumping on a trampoline because they do not contract mentally and physically. An academic, educator and former dancer discovered drumming at one of our courses. This woman in her fifties discovered the drum and took to it with a passion and it was a joy to see the exuberance rising through her as she played. Many teachers who have danced with us long to rewrite the curriculum and introduce new ways of teaching and learning, but they are often stymied by certain parents and the system. However, as more and more people discover new ways of being and seeing, these ways filter into every area of our lives. However, the individual cannot wait for the whole of society to wake up and give him or her permission to try a new way. The great artists and mystics went and did it for themselves and over time the others caught on. All of society expects us to be the same as everyone else and there is great resistance to change. Each one who finds his own beat begins to tune into the rhythm behind every living thing. When we are in rhythm we are steady and sure; what we need comes to us and we go towards what we need. When we try and walk or learn or live according to someone else's rhythm, we feel a little off, a little breathless and there is a strain around the heart. The muscles and tendons may try to pull one way, as our heads pull the other way, and the whole system is straining and bucking, as we are pulled away from our instinctive, spontaneous and natural impulses.

It is particularly important that we are in rhythm as we work so that we are working in harmony with our natural body rhythm. Antoinette describes this very well:

> A neighbour showed me not to push too hard when using the spade or the saw; not to clench my jaw and put effort into it, but to lean on the spade, to use the weight of it, to let the tool do the work. I learned from watching them, to bring a rhythm and pace into the task, not to be hasty, to find my balance on the ground, to square up to the task in hand.
>
> I learned to settle into my body, let out the tension in my breath. I witnessed the little rituals of a good working man. The quiet huff and puff and small whistling sigh that is the yoga of alignment of breath and body. The ritual of attunement. The preparation of tools, an eye to the weather, a sense of how long its going to take, how much will be done before lunch.
>
> The secret is in the preparation; and a realistic commitment to the job at hand. It requires a kind of settling-in to this body, this place, this task. It requires that things are set-up in such a way that I will be supported (with cups of tea) and not distracted from it by other tasks. When all that is in place, it is a

dance. I lean and move and rock and sway and pause to tackle any problem that arises. Once the rhythm establishes itself, and any aches or pains or residual impatience ease away, then the mind relaxes and stays softly focused on the job in hand, and an atmosphere of harmony and peace is created all around the person at work.

It is an atmosphere that is nourishing to the worker and to anyone who can hold their peace in the presence of it. A child becomes calm in the atmosphere of an older person working in this way.

When Tom came to see me first, he was very depressed. His body moved listlessly and his speech seemed to be sluggish and slow. He had a brilliant mind and had done really well in school and university. He was working as a psychotherapist and should have had a busy practice. However, Tom could not make money and his own depression was interfering with his work. When I tried to suggest different ways to him, he had a very well worked-out argument as to how these wouldn't work. It took quite a while to go below all that he knew and find some kind of simplicity. I noticed that all of the energy was up around his head and upper body but he had a good build and strong legs, as he had played football as a child. Over time, working with collage and spontaneous movement, it emerged that Tom had loved to watch old musicals when he was a child. As he spoke about Fred Astaire and Gene Kelly, I noticed his body becoming animated. His voice became lively and he lost the monotone he used when expounding one of his own theories about himself. Over time, Tom discovered the solution to his own problems. He needed to do more physically active work. He was brave enough to take up tap-dancing lessons and absolutely loved them. He also drummed and danced with me and found that he recaptured a lot of childlike spontaneity and playfulness. The more we worked with rhythm and also with solar plexus warrior-dancing, the more I saw his sense of humour and an intelligence that was now coming down into his feet and moving right through his body. He was often extremely funny when he moved, and had a natural comic talent. Slowly, Tom began to take steps to change his life. As he did this he became fearful, and once again I heard him attempting to analyse the child that he had been. I reminded him that the little boy did not understand all those big words, and, in order to feel safe, the child in him needed small things like reassurance, cuddles and a big blanket in which to wrap himself up when he felt afraid. Eventually, in order to recover fully, Tom took a sabbatical from his practice as a psychotherapist. During that year he continued with his dancing. Tom is now working with groups using dance and rhythm while drawing on his knowledge and experience as a psychotherapist. He has also danced in different amateur productions. I don't know if Tom will ever be a rich man, but he told me that he doesn't worry about money now as he is having too much fun.

What worked for Tom will not necessarily work for another person. Each person is dealing with different energy imbalances in the different chakras. However, most people can benefit from dancing because most disease arises from 'going out of rhythm' and an over identification with circular, addictive and habitual thinking.

Tribes

Working with earth and the base chakra, we divide the group into four tribes. The first rule of survival for the tribe is not competition but cooperation, working together to draw out each other's gifts. In this way the tribe is able to thrive creatively. Of course, being in a group brings up clan-of-origin tendencies and our survival issues in groups, but we are encouraging dancers to notice these and to begin to weave them into a creative expression within the tribe. All of the exercises, clues and devices we are using here are brought back to the tribe. Drawing on the experience of each member and their individual need for healing and creative inspiration, the tribe begins to forge an identity for itself

– a name or poem, a painting or symbol to represent it. This may happen by simply allowing a stream of consciousness from each member on their associations with the word 'earth'. All the time using devices that go below the surface thinker, who will tend to argue and try to compete and win within the tribe. When we sink deeper, tribal members are able to connect and begin to resonate with each other's rhythms. Even if there are personality clashes, these can be seen as fodder for creative expression.

Each member is finding a way to use their experience and how it relates to earth and tribal ritual. We can use any of the clues to create. For example, we might make a sculpture of roots, using our bodies and allowing them to twist, bend and entwine together. We can use photography to hone in on aspects of these body roots or we can paint them. As time progresses, the tribe may develop this into an expression of the healing needed in the roots by creating a song or a dance. Each member will be drawing on dreams they may be having, experiences among the trees and plants outside.

Another device we use is making huts or hiding places for the tribe to live in. This helps us to see what it is like to lie in a lair with 'family' and to notice what it feels like to have other tribes living nearby or further away.

Finally, all the tribes perform for each other with the intention of finding an expression of who 'we' are *now* in this body, in this tribe. Our intention is one of non-judgement and allowance. The results go even deeper as bodies begin to communicate in ways our surface minds can only guess at. Communication begins to take place in a much more authentic way, through muscle and bone, through poetry, song, movement and the use of earth props: stones, sticks, branches, bones, muck.

An expert in communication told me that the tribal song of the mother sung to her unborn baby and then sung by the whole tribe to that baby, at its birth and at key moments in that child's life, communicates to that child who it is and its tribal history much more efficiently than all of our history books, schools and computers. We begin to know this now as body knowledge.

One of our inspirations in Dancing the Rainbow was an African drum master who told us that in his language there is no such word as musician or non-musician because everyone is considered to be a musician and also a beginner. In that tribe, everyone dances and everyone sings, everyone paints and decorates as a part of daily life and as a way of expressing their spirituality and creativity. Also the aesthetic sense is not compromised because they have the most intricate and beautiful rhythms in the world, some of the most gifted dancers with beautiful posture, and singers whose voices are spontaneous and full of heart.

In older times in Ireland, when travellers from another tribe arrived at your door you did not engage them in long conversation. Firstly their feet were washed and then they were given food and a place to sleep. It was only after the body was cared for in this way that conversation could begin; the grounded comfort and safety of the body was the priority. When basic body needs are met with heart, we feel comforted and secure. All the luxury in the world cannot replace this grounded simplicity.

When we are dancing the roots, we sometimes have to cut away at them and trim them back. Sometimes we need to dig deep – down into the energetic roots – so we can replant, reshape and train them as we would a climbing plant. We work closely with nature to create from our roots instead of being pulled back by them or forced to grow in a way that is no longer healthy. In this way, each person finds a way to communicate and work deeply and creatively to heal the soul and the soul of the tribe.

In life, the people and tribes we are drawn to may be members of our soul tribes, and we can recognise them by the way they resonate with our rhythm and are drawn to our fire.

Exploration: Dancing the Roots

· If you can dance outside, you can let your bones imitate the roots of trees, the branches and twigs or the soft grasses by gently twisting your body into the shape of the root or swaying with the grasses and the wind.

· Notice the different shapes and the way each bone connects and each branch connects, sometimes in unexpected and innovative ways.

· You can stand with the palm of your hand against a tree. Notice the veins in your hand and sense into the veins in the tree.

· Dance the slow, deep dance of the roots by pushing downwards as if you were pushing into the earth.

· Then dance the lighter dance of the leaves by leading and moving from the extremities, the fingers and toes, and pushing and twisting upwards while the lower body pushes and twists downwards.

· Let your body become your own roots, feel how the roots push down into the earth and also strain to push up through her. Feel how they twist, bend and entwine as they push through the earth.

· Explore this fully with movement. You might wish to make sounds and expand this rooting into a dance.

· If you have someone to work with, you could take photographs of your body and the roots of the trees and use this in your collage. One of our dancers did this with a friend: they painted their bodies and took photos of a hand entwining with a branch, a face in the leaves and a body lying supine on a fallen tree.

· You can photograph roots, gather old pieces of gnarled wood and use these as inspiration for your dance. You could sit with a piece of bog oak and feel the texture of it in your own body. Or you can close your eyes and move your hands over it and smell it, gently letting it communicate with your bones. Let all of this inform your dance.

· Use earth, sand, stones, feathers or greenery to make something: a sandcastle with bridges, a dolmen, or whatever else comes. There is a great new wave of people making cob houses (houses made from the earth).

Exploration: Drawing on your Roots

- Put your feet into red paint and then place them on top of a sheet of paper, so the imprint of the soles of your feet is clearly marked on the paper. Enjoy the mess, but have a basin of warm water, soap and a towel to the ready and perhaps some soothing oils. You can ritualise this with a friend by blessing and honouring each other's feet and roots. Or you may prefer to work privately.

- The next day when the paint is dry, you can draw roots coming from the feet. You can then add words, photographs, pictures or paint. Do this gently and only when you feel ready and perhaps it is better done over time.

- If your family roots are too scary to look at right now or if you feel alienated from your family, put in pictures of a new tribe, one that would feel supportive and loving.

- You may feel an affinity to a tribe that might not be directly related to you, as far as you know. This could be a particular country or culture. Find pictures or simply put in words to acknowledge your connection to these people.

- When you are finished allow your body to move, but wait until the movements arise of their own accord and let your body find its own way.

- You can look at particular ways of your own family, tribe or clan, country of origin, regional traditions, religion, clothes. What is acceptable, to wear, say, etc.? Notice accents or languages.

- How do you feel when you step outside these conventions? What controlling influences are used in your clan, culture or family? How do you control your clan's reaction to you?

Una, one of our dancers, found it very hard to ground. She was mostly living in her head and could not really understand what we meant when we said things like 'come down into your legs'. She often suffered with panic attacks and a feeling of anxiety and foreboding. One day she got quite annoyed in the middle of the warm-up; she told me that she could not even feel her legs, so we began to do things to bring sensation down into the legs and buttocks: patting them, giving gentle little pinches, massaging her feet in a gentle and loving way. In this way she could bring more sensation and feeling down into her lower limbs.

Una really worked with this and also with the foot-painting and tracing her roots. Eventually her roots began to communicate with her through dreams and in smells and sensations. She had moved house a lot as a small child and had not had the opportunity to make friends. Her mother and father had found it hard to settle and had moved from one place to the next. The only steadying influence had been her grandmother whom she had lived with for long periods at a time. Looking back, she saw that her roots were back with her grandmother in that old house. Unfortunately, Una's grandmother died when she was five and she had never been able to grieve that loss or put words on it. Over time she danced the five-year-old she had been then and was surprised to see her feet curling up and away from the floor. She also noticed how she tried to lift her legs and feet off the floor. Una worked with collage and an earth altar to recreate the sense of home she had felt with her grandmother and she put a small amount of time aside every day to dance, sometimes simply when she was cleaning her house. At one stage in a private session it was very moving to see Una dance with her grandmother and to at last get a chance to say goodbye and to thank her for her love. Una then realised that despite having a home and family of her own, she had never been able to settle there and the house was something she inhabited rather than a place she called home.

Una worked with us over two years and by the end of that time she had moved house and was able to find a place she really liked by following her nose and trusting her own instincts. It was not an easy settling. She told me that like her parents, there were times she still felt like running away but little by little she was able to recapture her grandmother's way of settling in by the fire. Una had found it so hard to settle even to small household tasks. She was always planning ahead and worrying about the future, creating so much busyness outside of the house she spent very little time there. To her surprise, she found that one day she made no plans at all and little by little she was able to relax in her house with her family. Nobody else really noticed the difference in Una; to the outside world she was probably much the same but inside, where it mattered, Una was finally able to find rest and a sense of home. Her large root painting and collage hangs in the hallway with a photograph of her grandmother and some words of a song she used to sing, along with photographs of the different houses she lived in and one of children playing in the garden of her last house.

They say when the pupil is ready the teacher will appear. I am in the local pub waiting for the set-dancing to begin. The locals are gathering, and in he comes, my earthy man.

He is approaching sixty. He has been out with the horses all day. He talks about horses knowledgeably, laughs at the falls he has had. I would love to go horse riding, but am afraid I will fall. All that money I spent on osteopathy! He also drives a hearse and when I meet him on the road at the head of a funeral, he nods discreetly. It all mixes together now in the chat. 'I had a funeral Wednesday and then out with the horses Thursday.'

He cycles miles for charity, he goes sailing on the local lakes. He speaks knowledgeably about the local area. I am a blow-in and I don't know to where he is referring. I have been writing all day and I am a bit spaced and ungrounded.

We are called up and the music goes on. 'Right so, the Connemara.'

Circle and swing, then tops (top couples) advance and retire…circle around, home and swing.'

And we're off. He heads into it with a stamp of authority that grounds the group. Every so often he gives another stamp and tosses his head. His joints are loose and his arms and hands whoosh in time with the stamp. There's a batterin' goin' on. I can feel my feet coming down, the stamp calls me in. Whoo! Ancient, tribal, we find our feet. Stamp- stamp, flutter and stamp. Swinging round, every character comes to life. I can see them more clearly dancing than in any conversation we might have. There is a woman in her seventies dressed in beautiful colours with Dorothy's red shoes. She dances like a young, nervous pony. Then there are the bossy ones, heads forward.

'Not that way, House House.' (Dancing round the house)

Off we go, circling and swinging and my earthy man is stamping away. He's an Native American. He's an African elder. He's a Celt. The rhythm is in his bones. He is outdoors all the time. He is close to death and life every day, riding his horse, or sedately driving the hearse.

He 'shows the lady', circling his wife round the circle. The lady is gentle as the soft pastureland around us. A sense of place is what they have. Roots going deeply into this land.

Dancing with them, I absorb all of this. My own roots are tender and newly transferred from another place. I hold the scars of that uprooting; gently they begin to find a way through the stones of this place to find the dark limey earth that will hold them. Stamp. Stamp. The rhythm of the local accent, the hush of it, the cadence, soothes me.

Body as Home

Do you know your body? Are you kind to it? Can you touch it gently? Can you feel your body from the inside out? Are you aware of sensations? Can you feel your stiff neck, your rigid lower back, your tight jaw? Do you know when you are hungry? Are you always hungry? When are you tired? Are you often tired even though you have done very little physical work? Do you know what colours to wear and what your body would love; to dance or sing or have a massage or bathe in the river naked or cuddle up in a big fluffy blanket and be hugged? Do you like your body? Not in an image/fashion-conscious 'I'm a bit of all right', or 'I'm too sexy for my shirt' way; can you touch your body with tenderness and compassion? Would you like to? Do you ever feel angry? What do you do with that anger?

Any of the above questions could be used as a creative project. For example, you could make a collage exploring tenderness, compassion and comfort, or you could explore image and sexuality with photographs or through dance. You could simply take the word 'safety' and again take photographs or gather clothes, cloths, colours, little wooden boxes, nests – whatever strikes you. These questions bring us into the body again and again. Yes, we may think we are taking care of ourselves – but are we? Really?

Control and Image

In the base chakra, as in the throat chakra and solar plexus, we meet a big control centre. We can feel this in the bowel and lower back and also in the jaw, neck and upper back. There are two extremes: tight control and then losing control. When we objectify the body, we must control it and not allow it to communicate with us. We must keep it in order, keep up the mask, and we are terrified it will slip. We must make it look like an image of what we think it should be. In some cultures and countries, dancing and singing are forbidden. There was a time when dancing was forbidden in Ireland. Touch was also frowned on, and so dancers learned to dance with their arms held stiffly by their sides. This is all about control, and oppressive regimes throughout history have tried to control people's bodies, the way they sing, dance, write, paint, what they wear and the gods/goddesses they pray to. This oppressive regime may be functioning within our own bodies. There may be prison cells, walls and barriers within us; things we are not allowed to say; things we couldn't reveal; stories and songs that are still trapped behind the dams that were built in early childhood or the cultural prisons that existed when we were born or simply the ones we create for ourselves.

We may function in our bodies – go walking, play sports, eat, drink, make love, dance, ride a bike, even do yoga – and still not be in touch with the sensing body. We can still try to control the body by making it dance the way our minds or other people's have said that it should be done. For example, I may think that Irish dancing requires me to have ringlets and an ornate costume and enter competitions, but when my Irish body dances that is an Irish dance because my body is part of the landscape. Or you could push your body to become the perfect yogi and never come in contact with the effortless, soft sensing movement that comes from deep body knowledge and awareness.

You will notice sensations of hot and cold, pain and pleasure to the degree of how much you are in touch with your sensing body. Of course, body-oriented things like body exercise will help, but it is only by listening to the sensing body that we can learn its secrets. You can tell a lot by looking at someone's body. If you look from your conditioning, your likes and dislikes will get in the way of really seeing.

We have been taught that certain bodies are beautiful and others are not. It all depends on your family's beliefs, your culture, the ads on television and in magazines, or even what someone said to you in infant school. It seems that for some people in our culture now, injections into the forehead are required in order to be beautiful. In other cultures, they force huge amounts of milk down their throats because they want to be fat; fat is beautiful there. Our culture promotes breast implantations and the sucking of fat out of the thighs, cutting up the face and dragging the skin back over the face to make it tighter, and spending vast amounts of money on anti-ageing creams because ageing is considered ugly. You may dislike people with red hair because someone with red hair hit you once or did you some bad turn. In this way, your body can become a slave to your belief system.

I remember looking at myself in the mirror at about the age of eleven. I had just been watching the Miss World contest. I did a few toothy false smiles at myself and preened. Was I beautiful? I had teeth; they had teeth. I had masses of hair: that was good. Blue eyes; was that good? Maybe brown was better. Nose? Was I beautiful? What was beautiful? I went on to read the magazines or to listen to what other people said. Straight hair was in, so I was out. When curly hair came in I was in, but something else was wrong. So I began the rearranging of my looks according to what our advertising culture dictated. But first looks in the mirror can be pretty innocent. I remember observing myself in the mirror as a small child and looking at myself crying, noticing the downturn of my mouth and the tears without any judgement. I remember how I never saw my grandmother as old when I was a child. I noted her skin and white hair and false teeth without preconceptions. She was Granny, whom I loved to be near. My body sensed her out and felt safe and comforted.

If you look at a body in that way, without judgement, either good or bad, you will begin to see. If you can look, feel, touch and sense your own body in this way, you begin to know yourself. You are the only one you can truly know. Now you are able to step outside the narrow beliefs of your culture, as all great visionaries have been able to do. Now you can really begin to see and sense. You can look past the body image and into your soul.

Teaching young girls how to dance, I was horrified at how quickly rigidity took over from the soft, sensing body. In children as young as four years old, I felt the heaviness they were already learning to carry: heavy psychic and emotional energy they had absorbed from the atmosphere around them. It doesn't matter what education they get or how much they achieve, that heavy, energy body will weigh them down and create a psychic wall between them and life; the life inside and around them. It will create depression, low self-esteem and the need to relieve this psychic and emotional pain with drugs, drink or other addictions.

Years ago, children were overworked physically, but now we overwork the brain. Many children have never seen their food growing and do not know where it comes from. They love to work physically if it happens in a gentle, encouraging way; showing them how to bake brown bread, letting them cuddle and feed an animal. They love to build huts and create little homes. Most children love to make and create and this natural instinct can be built on. They are naturally physical and playful; movement and exercise is a part of what they do, and what they can teach adults to do if they are given the space and unstructured time simply to play. When children have the experience of growing food and herbs and then preparing and cooking them, they learn in their bodies how much things cost in physical energy. Knowing how our natural food is grown keeps us grounded and we don't waste energy. We honour the earth, the animals and our own bodies. Any work with natural materials can begin to attune us with this soft, undulating, earthy body. This heals the fear and brings us comfort and security.

How can we begin to understand our body? Not by twisting it and trying to make it behave, or pounding it into shape or looking at bits of it under a microscope. We can understand and know the body by getting to know it just as we would a new friend.

Whether we admit it or not, the landscape around us affects our bodies and our health. Time spent in lush, untainted nature brings one home and eases mind and body. Control and image then begin to dissolve into nature's dance and simply cease to exist. It is the same if we listen to music or dance until we sweat; eventually the controlling thoughts let go and for a time we are free.

It takes great courage to follow the desire of your heart; to use your feet, putting one in front of the other, each step leading you. Staying present and taking the next step reveals the next one: even when our old panic and fear rears up to tell us it is impractical and that we need to organise our pensions, not dream in colours.

The trick is to take that first step no matter what it is. Picking up the phone to ring someone who can help or buying a little notebook and some coloured pens: these are practical steps. We also need to check that we are taking these steps to fulfil our own life purpose, not what we *think* we should do. If the fear escalates and we find that we are pushing against insurmountable obstacles, then we may not be going the right way or the timing is wrong. Often, we need to learn something before we move on. Perhaps we need to learn more about money management if no one ever taught us and it was always a scary subject. Perhaps we need to feel a sense of home before we can expand out into the world. Mostly we need to come home to the soft, sensing body and be as fully present as we can be, so that fear is not pushing us forward.

It takes time to come into the rhythm of life, to trust that rhythm, not to push and not to hang back. Gently take the fear and make a dance or a poem from it; listen to it, what is the fear trying to say? What kind of a dance would this fear create?

The roots of the body can take many years to heal and yet, in a moment, when we are dancing or resting in stillness, we are able to come to a place of complete acceptance and freedom. If you dance the roots you can become aware of the issues that can be triggered in the base and what movements worked best for you before. I have spent many years healing my relationships with my roots and with the earth and I now understand that we can return to base and make it safe, see that we can build our own houses, and grow our own vegetables. We may choose not to, but the fact that we can means we are not being run by fear of authority figures who own the land, our homes, our bodies, our creativity and our time. See that your body is your home and you can dance your dreams and weed out and clear energy that is no longer useful in your body and your life. You can plant the seeds for fresh new growth. If you use these explorations well, there is no doubt that you will heal old issues and generate greater creative freedom within yourself and in your life.

Survival

Nature has endowed nearly all living creatures with very similar nervous system responses to the threat of danger. However, of all species, there is only one that routinely develops long-term, traumatic after effects – the human. The only time we see similar effects in other animals is when they are domesticated or consistently subjected to stressful conditions in controlled laboratory environments. In these cases, they develop acute and chronic traumatic reactions.

Peter A. Levine, *Waking the Tiger*

Flight

When faced with the threat of danger, there is a rush of adrenalin and the energy flows to the parts of the body that need to act. You can feel cold or hot when this happens. If you can physically fight, the body uses this build-up of energy. If you can run, it also has the chance to use the energy. If not, you freeze, and even then, if you survive the threat, your body will find ways to use the surplus energy. However, when we are experiencing fight or flight because we are afraid of something that happened in our past, we can be in a constant state of anxiety, with the adrenals over-functioning until we eventually begin to experience chronic stress and burn out. The above quote is from Peter Levine's book which describes his work with trauma and gives detailed and simple instructions on what to do in traumatic situations so the body can access its own natural healing. This knowledge is essential and could be taught in schools as the distress created by untreated trauma is great indeed.

One of my teachers described to me how, after visiting the dentist, she goes to the toilets and allows her body to shake and yawn, and then when she comes home she lies down to rest. She has spent so long working with trauma she knows now how to release it from her body safely and easily. This is very good advice, as the body will then naturally heal from the shock of the tooth removal. However, if the body does not heal naturally, strange aches and pains can be felt for days afterwards and one could feel low, tired or anxious.

There are other ways, for example kinesiology, touch for health, that has simple but profound ways of releasing old frozen trauma from anywhere in the body, including the internal organs.

In peer-counselling groups, I watched people speak about traumatic situations that happened years before. As they spoke, their bodies would begin to shake and they would begin to yawn. They were taught to take notice of what the body needed to do to release and heal, instead of getting caught up in the story. Watching the body heal in this way was invigorating, a living theatre. When we cannot work through our emotions, we use something to change them – food, substance or a behaviour – and this can become addictive.

When as a child I was put in hospital, I submitted to everything and envied children who screamed and ran after their mothers. I was a nice little girl and did what I was told. If I did not like something I played dead, left my body, bypassed my brain altogether and spaced out; this was the only way I could flee. Now, faced with a similar frightening situation, I may involuntarily do the same thing; because my body is triggered in this way I am not free. This is what psychotherapists call dissociation from one's own body. It's a great word – dissociation. In her book *Getting our Bodies Back*, Christine Caldwell describes beautifully how we develop addictive body movements that we use in order to dissociate, for example habitual nose rubbing.

> Our bodies are clever. Like children in a fairy tale they leave
> a trail of breadcrumbs to help them find their way back out
> of the dark forest. Our bodies use movement habits to mark
> the spot where we check out. Like a breadcrumb trail, these
> gestures enable us to trace our way home.
>
> Christine Caldwell, *Getting our Bodies Back*

I think it is particularly sensitive to use the image of a child in a fairy tale leaving a trail of breadcrumbs to help them find their way back out of the dark forest because that is exactly what it has felt like to me, and to have a loving other help me make sense of these chronic movement habits and skilfully help me to find their source has been the most empowering and freeing experience I have ever had.

As I come back into my body then, I meet these old movement habits, sensations, the incomplete experience lodged somewhere in my body memory. If I stay with these sensations without thinking, my body will begin to heal itself. I will shake or begin to yawn or even cry or explore the movements very slowly in a funny little dance. Unfortunately, as the fear escalates I will find myself trying to *think* my way out of it, a twisted version of the impulse to run. Even thinking positively is a way I try to escape the sensations. Or I may run away from a situation or person when it is inappropriate to do so because I am feeling all of those old impulses to flee still lodged somewhere in my body, but beginning now to melt and release. Or I will want to attack someone, either myself or someone else as I 'act out the old trauma'. In the midst of all of this, because of old trauma arising, I will not be able to think straight. Confused thoughts will battle it out as the old emotions and sensations surface and I may become frozen, unable to take any action at all. If I can begin to move, even in a small way, and begin to use these habitual movements more consciously, they can lead me to a more authentic expression of my deeper truth.

Whenever we dance, we visit these old survival fears with tribal and family issues erupting. At the beginning of one of our courses we were in a beautiful house with gorgeous grounds. We had gone to great trouble to decorate the room and to make it welcoming for the people who gathered, all strangers to each other. Yet the fear was icy in the room. The place reminded some people of old boarding schools; someone else thought there was not going to be anything to eat because she had mistimed the tea. There was a bit of panic over the lack of towels. You could see by people's bodies that they were preparing to flee or have a row with us – fight or flight – or stay physically but space out of the body and leave in that way. There were big survival fears over apparently small things. If I had tried to point this out to the group, it would not have worked. I have tried this before, but the fearful thinker immediately gives me an argument. Instead we begin with dance and movement.

First of all, we connect to the instinctive animal in us and begin by checking out what is happening in the body by slowly moving through the body and acknowledging the sensations there. We breathe into the fear and let it inform our movements and then we begin to sniff around and explore the space in a leisurely way. The more we use these simple physical movements, the easier it is to cope with these fears. As the group grounds, they are able to move more freely, and have a greater sense of space and their relationship to the other bodies in the room. When the body feels grounded and safe, then you can begin to create the dances which flow easily.

This group was eventually able to laugh at their own fears, but they were also able to trace the roots of these fears and use them in their tribal dances. They would also know that these fears arise quite naturally when we enter a new situation. Any animal left out of a car in a strange place will sniff the place out and the people in it before he settles to eat or rest.

Coming into a new group/tribe or experience, we need to ground our fear. First of all we need to come more fully into the body while also noticing our judgemental thoughts: these judgements are trying to protect us, but, in fact, if we are in real, immediate danger, thinking is not going to help us. We have been taught to think instead of move. As children we learn rules of behaviour that inhibit our natural instincts. The thinking we used then rises up inappropriately to try and help us in a new situation.

Antoinette often speaks about how boring she found adults when she was a child because they seemed just to sit around all the time talking and she decided even then that when she was grown up she would still move around and play. As we get older we can become afraid of playing, especially with new people. We can waste a lot of time looking for something or someone to pin the fear on. We cannot see clearly because we are approaching a new experience, and our thoughts are trying to make it familiar by associating it with past experiences, usually frightening ones. This new experience may be something expansive and exciting and we need to be able to open our hearts and minds so that we can let it in and enjoy it. However, we may need to acknowledge our fears first and be gentle with the past. For example, Anna was going on a romantic weekend away with her new partner; his treat. As the day for departure neared, she became nauseous and her body was going hot then cold. The beginnings of flu, she thought, and worried about not being able to go, or perhaps experiencing a panic attack when she was there. I asked her what this trip was reminding her of and she said, 'I don't know.' 'Well, if it was to remind you of something, what would it be?' Immediately she named a former boyfriend and a holiday they had had when she was seventeen. Young and inexperienced, this had not been a good holiday for many reasons. Now, years later, that old experience was returning to haunt her but in a way that she couldn't even relate to. She took time to talk to the seventeen-year-old she had been and also to listen. The next morning, out of the blue, the former boyfriend rang for a friendly chat, so now she got to re-experience this old trauma and resolve it in the present. All the physical symptoms disappeared immediately and she had a gentle, romantic time with her new partner.

Returning to the Body – Soul Retrieval

We begin to breathe into the body, come down into the feet and notice if the body is trembling. We acknowledge our movements, and, at the same time, provide the safe ground for the body to express itself gently and easily.

I remember one man in the room with a crowd of women, his teeth chattering and his body shaking with fear. He had come to dance and he had to go through all this fear so he could do something he really wanted to do. At every moment I was afraid he would run out of the door. I acknowledged his fear and encouraged him to let the shaking move through his body, I also acknowledged how brave he was to be following his creative dreams. Afterwards, he told me that the child in him felt affirmed, he had always wanted to dance but had been too scared as a child to go down to the local dance class which was full of girls. He really was very tuned into his body, because at least he was shaking and his teeth were chattering instead of being masked by a cool exterior personality. Because the fear was right there, he was able to express this fear through his dance, and the group, seeing their fear mirrored in his, immediately took to him and welcomed him in.

When we accept our bodies just the way they are and allow those bodies to express their experience creatively, it allows a bigger story to be told. A good actor needs to be able to express human emotion in face and body movement. A dancer needs this ability even more, and yet our bodies are telling secret stories of which we are not even aware. I remember the day that my body-based therapist pointed out that even though I was professing fond love for someone I was involved with at the time, my left hand was clenched into a fist. This was a missing clue to my story, this unknown anger. Without access to these hidden sensations and emotions, I can be stifled creatively and in my relationships. Even if I am practising a spiritual discipline, I may notice my surface thoughts but the surface thoughts are hiding the deeper tendencies and beliefs. It is these deeper tendencies that are creating my experiences. There are rivers of mystery running through the clay of this body. As I began to experience the emotions and sensations fully, I began to create from the naked integrity of my body's truth. This can be scary and it can be exhilarating and it is a way to find true freedom.

So we reach and stretch and breathe and let the fear run through the body. We become animals checking the place out, sniffing round and sniffing each other. The old fear of the instinctual comes up as we grunt and groan and moan and let out the sound of that fear. This in itself can be frightening because we only allow our voices to make little polite sounds. When we explore all the sounds and all the movements, we give birth to a wild, earthy dancer.

We can become very detached from our body's natural functions and be very prissy about them. That cuts us off from our life force. When we cut off from the life force, we are forced up into the thinker: always trying to think or analyse our way out of trouble. Thinking and talking about the past, our problems or the future, we are unable to push our feet down into the earth and be here now. Or we can be very creative and forget to eat or sleep. It is as if parts of the soul are detached from other parts and from the roots of our being. Our bodily functions are ignored or perhaps not even felt. Often there is a striving for some spiritual or intellectual ideal that does not acknowledge the lower body. In its extreme, this leads to a need to eradicate all that does not fit in with the mind's idea of what is good, clean or spiritual: religious wars; racism; mass murder; violence; petty gossip; judging and making other people our scapegoats. So much pain is visited on each other in the name of a god or a perceived truth.

Or we become totally tied up in survival fears, worrying about money, trying to feel secure inside by having enough on the outside.

Feet to the ground: that is the key here, feet to the ground and being able to stand on your own two feet. Dancing the colours, I see people fall to the ground, immobilised, unable to move, stuck. If they simply experience what it feels like to be stuck and find a simple gesture or position to express that then the body and mind finds a way to digest and integrate this information. Finds a new way of being and moving. If you let your body be and it gets safe to be like that, you change.

On we go dancing, stamping the rhythm with our feet, clapping it, drumming it. We have danced around people who were lying there. One man used to lie in the middle of the floor with a towel wrapped around his head to test the instruction 'move or don't move whatever way you like'. We danced around him and jumped over him.

When I am dancing, children often come and look in the doorway, but even when invited they will not join in. Wise little beings, they watch and wait and then, when it feels safe, in they come.

It is the same with all the parts of our soul: the shy child within, the angry one, the old wise shaman who was ridiculed for his beliefs, the healer woman who was killed because she loved nature, the hunted wild animal. They may feel uncomfortable and unable to join in. They stay there and wait and eventually, with a bit of luck, they begin to move stiffly, warily, clumsily, repetitively, finding their way, watching the other dancers. Like a child learns by watching its mother and absorbing the way she moves, learning by imitation and exploration and also listening. In this way we begin to understand how other people experience their physical reality and our bodies can learn how to move differently or more easily. No one interferes, and their bodies show them it is now safe to move, to shake, to be scared, to get hot and cold, to cry, to sweat, to not do any of that, and the miracle of the body that can hold and contain all of this.

If the body needs to shake, we dance that shaking; let it become the dance. If we need to flee, we can run and see what that feels like or we can play fight. The energy will shift and move and begin to dissolve. Eventually there is no space between the movement of body and the mind. I am observing, I am observing, and then magically I am it. I am the dance and there are no thoughts, no emotions; all the disparate parts of me enjoying the sensation of my body moving this way and that, fully in the now.

Funny, gentle things can happen that help us with our creative process if we are alert to any signs or messages coming to us in the weeks before or after we have been dancing; there are gangs of angels helping us in every way and some of those angels are our ancestors who understand all too well what we are here to do.

Karen was a dancer who had an abusive father. Because of his treatment, she had severe learning difficulties. When he was shouting at her over her homework she shut off her hearing and eventually when he pushed her over she fell and damaged her eyes. She suffered with eye problems and dizzy spells as well as experiencing a lot of pain in her body. Karen was attending an insightful therapist who encouraged her to attend the DTR course. She had not done any bodywork before, as it was too painful, and we encouraged her to trust her own body and not push herself when she was dancing. Karen loved to dance even though at first her movements were quite limited and often jerky. She had been haunted by her memories for so long but in the dance she found that she was relatively free of them, even though her body was actually leading her towards them. Over a few years, I watched Karen's progress. Because she loved the dance she eventually began to give dance workshops, even though her own body was in pain and she could not demonstrate the movements she wanted from her class. She found ingenious ways around this. She would demonstrate her own restricted movement and encourage her dancers to come to the edge of their own restriction and dance from there. Because she was so open about her own body, other people enjoyed her classes. They felt comfortable to show what they saw were their own barriers to dance and movement and from there all the other ways they felt restricted in their lives. Eventually Karen wanted to expand her dance classes and train as a body-based psychotherapist as well. In order to do that, she had to face her learning difficulties and she did this step by step, finding people who could help and guide her. She couldn't do this as a child, but now, as an adult finding her own feet, she could get the help she needed. Developmentally, this made sense because before she could face these learning difficulties she needed to feel some kind of safety in her own body. Karen had a gifted therapist, but she could not have done what she did without courage. Karen told me that she finds her courage when she dances because slowly she has found a deep compassion for the way her body has survived and healed.

When we allow our bodies to be true, they express our pain and our joy and our soul's journey to this place, this moment. It is a privilege to witness this living art in every twisted shape, in every cry, and in the rhythm that rises up from the earth and surges through the fear, transmuting it and grounding this groundless fear through the conductor of the body. The healing takes place in the body first and it is only later that the thinking comes into line with this new way of being.

Freezing and Creative Blocks

Another dancer rang me, as she was getting ready to lead a dance workshop. Unfortunately she kept getting sick and found that she was unable to move or organise herself for the work. When she thought of cancelling she started to feel better, but when she tried to imagine giving the workshop and preparing tapes, etc., she froze. I could pick up her intense fear on the telephone and she was relieved to have it named as fear as her thoughts were masking the fear by trying to justify backing out of the workshop. She was saying that she didn't feel excited anymore about the work and maybe it wasn't really for her. Of course we can't feel enthused about our creative inspirations all the time; eventually it becomes work, the hard labour of bringing something into form. We worked together on the phone and with a body visualisation. I also gave her a recipe that was handed on to me from Mo Griffiths, an elder who teaches and passes on the knowledge of the flower essences discovered by Edward Bach. This is an excellent support for freezing fear. The flower essences seem to work directly with the nervous system, and help the body not to contract rigidly when faced with an experience that either triggers an old fear that immobilises us or when we are about to move beyond our comfort zone and do something powerful. It's not that it fixes the fear, but it softens the resistance and helps us to filter, work through and integrate it. I got another call from this DTR teacher on Monday. She had taken the remedy and had gone to the workshop. She used her own fear as the theme for her workshop and encouraged the participants to explore their creative dreams and the fears that were holding them back. They then went on to dance that and find a creative expression for that fear. Instead of polarising the fear and the creativity, this teacher now saw that it was part of it. The workshop had gone really well. Over the phone I could hear her voice was coming from down deep in her body; she sounded relaxed and in rhythm with her life and her life purpose.

Jane was a good writer who had published short stories and then she stopped. During the DTR course she slowly began to write again, mainly after dancing and moving. Something freed up in her and the words began to come again. After a while she began to write about what happened to her around the time she stopped writing. She had written some really sensitive stuff in her diary about her past, and her ex-husband had used her diaries in court as a way of trying to prove that she was unfit to parent her children. Even though the diaries were not allowed as any kind of evidence, the shock of having her private writing read and used against her in such a way had caused the writer in Jane to freeze. At the time, she had worked through this and felt that the writing was a phase in her life that was now over. The deeper truth was that the writer was very hurt and also afraid to speak – frozen, immobilised and silenced. When her body began to move, something shifted and she began to write again. At first, the writing was very private and Jane created an altar in her own bedroom where she put her diaries, wrapped in pink and gold muslin and ribbons, signifying the sacredness and privacy of her work. After some time she began to publish poems again and then the writing took a turn and she began to write songs.

Our creativity is such a gentle, private process; it needs time to be nurtured and encouraged. We need space to access our deepest truths and to heal any roots that have been damaged, so we can grow the plant of our creative project to full maturity until it is strong enough to stand on its own. There is no point trying to push or force our bodies to do this with the mental body because sometimes the body has skipped over a developmental stage and is literally unable to put one foot in front of the other in order to go towards something. Or we may even be unable to put out a hand to reach for something the body needs. It only makes the situation worse if we try and bully ourselves to do something. Working with gentleness and ease allows the body time to access the movements and the support needed to advance, sometimes to retreat, and sometimes to simply accept the present moment exactly as it is.

Passion

The inspirational book, *A Course in Miracles*, says that even slight irritation is a mask over killing rage. Contacting that rage, even suspecting that it is there, can be scary and life-changing. We may be afraid because that rage has been turned inwards and vented on ourselves and on our physical bodies in all sorts of ways: not giving ourselves enough time to be alone or to do what we want to do, or not allowing time to take loving care of our bodies. We become unable to create or live our lives fully because we have been hurt or put down. We keep ourselves occupied by watching telly, talking, eating, cleaning, sleeping, avoiding.

We may begin to have backache, feel weak or have panic attacks as we turn it back in on ourselves. We may become sick or chronically tired, constipated, weak in the legs and hips, develop stiff knees and hips, fear of moving, heavy tiredness, blood pressure imbalances, non-stop smoking or eating or exercising, cutting the body, spacing out, criticising and putting ourselves and others down, making others into scapegoats with perfectionist thinking and little attacks. We may become addicted to spiritual or addictive highs and find ourselves unable to cope with ordinary life. Or we may lie in bed feeling helpless, with strange aches and pains in our bodies. These are just some of the ways our creative passion twists and turns.

When Jean came to see me first she found it hard to walk up the stairs to the dance studio I was working in. She had to hold the rail and go up one step at a time, her face contorting in pain. She had had several operations on her spine and doctors were burning the nerves in her spine to alleviate some of the dreadful pain she was experiencing day and night. I was not very experienced working with a dancer with this degree of pain and I was not quite sure how I was going to be of any use to Jean. I simply outlined the ways I had worked with my own physical and emotional pain, being careful to explain that the physical pain had not been so intense and that I did not have back operations to take into the equation. I also told her that she needed to be very careful how she moved that body. But Jean seemed to jump at the chance of being able to find creative ways to express her physical pain. She was in such pain that all her defences were down. Jean is a very gentle woman, religious and dedicated to her family. In the dance studio she became a screaming virago. At first she was afraid that she would act out this rage in her life, but after a while she began to experience relief from the pain. She was particularly angry at the Catholic church because one of the clergy had abused her over a number of years when she was a child. I just sat there and let her get on with it. I gave her some pointers about the spine and the connection to her tail and her nose. I also encouraged her to stay grounded through her legs, feet and hands so that the rage did not spin her off and out of her body. Her body did the rest. She followed the sensations in her lovely, sensitive body and she moved the way it led her. Eventually it led her up onto her feet and she created beautiful, passionate dances. At that time I was young and enthusiastic about how dance could free up the body and the creative soul. But even I found it unbelievable that within months of working weekly with movement, this woman was walking easily up the stairs. For other people it may not ever work like that because the physical damage is so severe, but for Jean it worked. A life-time's rage was in that spine. Long before physical and sexual abuse within the Catholic church had been revealed in the media and when it was still a dark secret within the Irish psyche, Jean used the power of her rage to write one letter every week to the Catholic church. She told her story and asked what they were going to do about it. Eventually they replied.

In dance workshops I have watched people prostrate on the ground and felt the heavy atmosphere in the room. We go with the exhaustion, we feel it, allow it to pin us to the ground. This deep, unconscious stuff can send you to sleep, and it is heavy, turgid, and drags the face and eyes down. We might begin by gently pushing cushions at each other or by trudging around the room – heavy, heavy, weighed down. The weight of the past pressing down on the head and shoulders, all those bloody thoughts. Then eventually the heaviness lifts and we snarl and fight and roar. All of this is done in a light, playful way, but there is no mistaking it. Men and women become tribal; their feet remember old warrior dances. We let go and let the body take over, but with awareness and the intention of healing.

Remember that blue is the complementary colour to red. Red is warming and blue is cooling. If you are feeling a lot of rage or very hot in your body, dance the base but breathe in blue and surround your self with the cooler blue colours. You can also use turquoise and pink to soften the impact of old rage so that it releases through the body gently and easily.

Instinct

The fear in the base chakra is different from the fear in the other chakras. The fear in the sacral centre is related to emotions and relationships and fear of retriggering old hurts or being hurt. The fear in the solar plexus is the fear of the mind and the thoughts and sometimes fear of losing our opinions or our belief system and ego identity, sometimes fear of our own power and authority. The fear in the heart is mysterious and connected to our relationship with love on every level. The fear in the throat is tied up with being able to express ourselves truthfully on every level. The fear in the third eye is often tied up with old superstition and religious abuse. The fear in the crown can be huge because it relates to spiritual power. The fear in the base chakra at its most natural is a 'shit-yourself' fear. For example, if a wild animal came into your sitting room you would not sit there thinking about it; hopefully your legs would move faster than your thoughts.

Antoinette and I were walking in the countryside and I was thinking, 'This is nice, now we will go up to the wood and I will sink into the present moment.' Antoinette's voice was the first warning, 'Eh, should they b-b-b-eee here…?' A herd of bullocks, wild after being shut up all winter, were coming aggressively towards the dog and us. Eventually they were chasing the dog and we were nearly flattened in the stampede. As they came towards us, Antoinette took up a stick and said to me, 'Don't show fear.' Too Late! Talk about coming into the present moment! I tried to manoeuvre my body across the lumpy ground and out of the way. At one stage I tried to hide behind a tree and then realised they could get round it. All the time, say ten minutes, when this was going on, there were no thoughts, just bowel sensations and running. Antoinette stayed and fought with her stick; I took flight and left her there! In that moment I was no hero because the dog kept running towards me with the bullocks after her. It was every man for himself.

Afterwards, shaking and laughing and checking out injuries, mostly to clothes that had caught on barbed wire, we wanted to talk about it and complain and look for justice by finding out who was responsible for the bullocks' behaviour. The dog was exhilarated from the chase, tongue hanging out, almost laughing at the good of it. However, I noticed afterwards that when I walked in country fields I had a residual fear in my body. My belly tightened, my throat felt dry and I felt a desire to run. I decided I would dance this, letting my body go with these sensations. This finally resolved itself when a herd of bullocks came into my garden; there came a quick flashing image of the havoc they were going to cause to the lawn and the new little trees. I went thundering out the door waving a sweeping brush at them; they were on my territory now and they knew it. They galloped heavily away. Studying animals and being aware of their instincts makes us more alert. We can feel when we are in their territory and sense their reactions to us and how we can respond instinctively to them. We can also notice this instinct at work when we are in new places, with new people or in another person's house. We can notice how our behaviour might change in order to fit in with theirs or we might notice how we feel when they are in our house or in our country: not to act inappropriately on these instincts, but certainly to honour them and allow them to shift and change. Jan Fennel's book, *The Dog Listener*, teaches so much about the behaviour of pack animals. By reading it, we can also understand that our own instincts need to be honoured. Sometimes people say, 'But surely we will all end up acting like animals with no morals at all?' However, animals in the wild work from pure instinctual intelligence and this has its own integrity. Human cruelty has a much bigger range, where the power of imagination and reflection is often used to torture not only ourselves, but the earth and all that live on it. When we bring the intelligence of a still mind, together with the instinctual intelligence in the body, we work in harmony with nature not against her.

Smell

A Dancing the Rainbow student from South Africa was describing an incident where he was standing by a waterfall and began to notice that his little dog was holding his head up and sniffing the air. He was glad he had he noticed because then he smelt something himself; the smell of rotting meat in a leopard's teeth, and the heavy smell of wild animal. He was out of there fast. His dog's sense of smell saved him here.

This instinct feels different to us now because it has been tied into the thoughts and that can put us off the scent. Sometimes in my car I get a bowel sensation and I slow down; sure enough there is usually some driver coming at high speed halfway over the road. The more we get in touch with our roots, the more this essential instinct of fear/attack or stand your ground gets a chance to protect us. If we lose our instinct we die, even if we are still walking around working and doing, some essential life force is missing.

It is not often that I would meet such a clear, clean impulse of fight or flight as I did in the woods that day when we were chased by the bullocks. Unfortunately our bodies are bogged down with old, frozen or unassimilated wounds and sometimes we do not know what we are afraid of. Even so, the instinct is still there and the body knows how to heal itself. For example, at a workshop recently I could feel the muscles in my body tight and contracted, my emotions were in turmoil, my head distressed and confused and I was rubbing my nose and ear in a distressed way. I looked behind me and saw Antoinette playing with home-made dough and flour. She was patting it with her floury hands, cutting it and shaping it. Immediately I felt a calmness seep into my body. Everything became safe as instinctively I edged over and began to pat and play, conscious that no one was going to shout at me. I drew comfort from this simple thing; the smell of the dough and the simple rhythm of Antoinette's hands as she shaped it. It was enough; by some alchemy these moments can heal years of fear. There is no need then to flee or fight and the warm animal body can come to rest.

A midwife who worked with native peoples says that she knows how far along the labour is by the smell. Other women can tell when they are ovulating by the smell and they can smell illness coming from their children before they actually become unwell. Another man clears old stale energy from houses and land and tells me that he can smell it out. Our sense of smell is a powerful tool for survival and health and immediately links us with our instinctive intelligence.

One of our dancers had a very poor sense of smell and this affected her sense of taste. She had had this condition and accompanying nasal problems from the time she was a child. After dancing her roots she slowly began to recover her sense of smell. Sometimes she found this very hard, especially when the smells were ones she associated with unpleasant memories from which she wanted to recoil. However, over time she stayed with it and, by going with it and feeling all the sensations associated with the event, it eventually became just another memory instead of a physical trauma that could be triggered by smell.

The sense of smell is tied in with the sense of sight and hearing. It is possible to smell, hear and even taste colour and energy. When we block our senses because of unpleasant or threatening events, we also block our vitality and our energy. Of course we need to unblock slowly and gently and without frightening ourselves again. This can be done subtly and creatively with the help of nature and our own creative nature.

Body Intelligence

When animals experience life-threatening events, they quickly move beyond the initial shock reaction and recover. Their reactions are time-limited and do not become chronic. Observing this behaviour can give us an understanding of our own instinctual ability to successfully overcome trauma. We can also learn more about how not to interfere with our instincts.

Peter A. Levine

The body is fascinating to me, especially the clean, animal body. Once I realised I was an animal with fairly primitive but accurate instincts, I could get to the truth behind the chatterbox in my head. I could also get to the instinctual, intelligent nature within my body.

I found it was best to follow the intelligence in my own body rather than interpret it with what someone else had discovered. I also found that if I did not try to force myself to do things when I was not ready, my body's intelligence would find a way gently to reveal where I was stuck. Sometimes my body found the most creative ways to heal itself and, if I trusted my body, I discovered a rhythm that was at one with the rhythm of the earth. For example, if I tried to advertise a workshop before the energy was with me, there would be no response or a response that was as half-hearted or ungrounded as I was feeling. If I waited until my idea had form and shape with good strong roots, people responded with enthusiasm and energy. With creative projects I noticed that if I was anxious or tired but had a deadline, I needed to trust my body first and not push for the deadline. I would give my body attention, rest and quiet. If I just gave my body one hour or even five minutes attention, it saved so much energy because then I wouldn't be trying to push through something, I would be working with it and waiting for the next wave of energy to catch me and carry me along, just like a mother giving birth who waits for the contraction before she pushes. In this way my tasks would be completed in a rhythmic and joyful way. Of course sometimes I tried to push and control and sometimes other people tried to push and control me. However, as my body got healthier I would take the time to lie down and rest or move and dance and it always rewarded me. Things take less time and effort because the whole body system is working in harmony. We can become like the wild animals, apparently dozing, resting, dawdling, but, when the time is right, leaping with grace and accuracy. We also get staying power, the ability to stay with the job in hand without trying to escape from the present.

When we wake up in the morning we may have become ungrounded during the night, and our thoughts and fears can be magnified. Instead of jumping out of bed to obey these fear voices, put them on hold for a moment and breathe. I find it helpful to make contact with my animals by petting or feeding them; this grounds me. Or else I write out all the worries and thoughts and put a colour round them and then do some simple and gentle movement work. Elaine puts on the kettle and, by performing what she calls 'a menial task' like cleaning out the fire and emptying the ashes outside, she gets a chance to take in the day and connect with the elements; then she has her tea. Don roasts seeds for his porridge and does a tribal dance on his way to the shower. Eleanor rubs in oils in front of the fire and then does the rainbow warm-up. David touches and smells his artwork. So when I am giving you suggestions of ways to work, these are clues to help you find your own ways rather than something to be followed mechanically. These are clues and tools that may help; the real intelligence is within you and comes behind your breath and heartbeat. However, habitual thoughts often try to stop us moving. In all the time we have been working, we have never found that dancing was a mistake, even when we did not want to get up and move or we wanted to go on talking. Once we had danced and moved, even if it were only for a few minutes, we all agreed afterwards that we felt much better.

Healing our Roots

The following extract is from a very strong dream Joanne, a trainer with DTR, had as she danced and healed her instinctual body and her roots.

> Last night in my dream, I was brought back to my ancestral house, the house of my father's people, and his people before him, and his people before him; the house built by my male ancestors, three generations ago, on the site, in the kingdom, between the fairy fort and the castle of O'Connor, underneath the sky of *Cnoc an Oir*. I was brought back through time to the beginning. The shed was different, so, so mucky, and my feet were sinking in deep, wet, sludging earth. Wild people came out of the cow sheds – gypsies, fierce and scary looking – they regarded us, we regarded them, but we and they continued on our ways. They were supposed to be there, with their ruddy faces red and weather-beaten, and their wild hair. The house was in total ruin and decay, walls rotted, damp, beautiful colours, almost bare of furniture, walls pale blue, white, cream, cool and cold. I looked in, scared, through each doorway from the hall: first the little bedroom on the left, my room, where I slept on the bed made of cardboard boxes, where my dog rusty would jump in on me; the room with the hatch into Granny's bedroom; the spooky bedroom, the bedroom that was deep and secretive as a cave, where little girls only peeked in from the door, the creepy, freaky old black scroll calendar and crucifix, the black, deep trunk, the old lone iron bed deep in the cave, the emptiness, the room that always seemed temporary, non-permanent, as if my Granny was only visiting there.

This is a lovely account of that dream-like state where old root issues rise up to consciousness. In these dreams or visions, our way is intimated to us and we can gain new understanding about who we are and where we have come from. Sometimes we meet long-lost relatives in our dreams and in our lives. You will also find old issues coming up again and again, if you are making changes in your life, as you let go of old ways of being, or as old friends or relationships move on. When this happens, it is good to come back and read about and dance with the roots and the instinctual body. Each time we do this our roots become stronger and we are able to move with the wind without collapsing. Another wonderful result of doing this work is that your children will benefit. As you heal your own roots and body, remember that they are also growing from these roots so their lives heal as well. Also, by some trick of time and place, you are healing the roots of your family, your parents, grandparents and great-grandparents. The sap moves from the deepest roots to the smallest twigs, and it returns from the small twigs back down into the roots.

As you dance and transform your body and therefore the roots of all people – for we are all connected through our roots – I honour you, your bones and the bones of your ancestors.

Invitation to Dance

I invite you now to use these clues/attributes and the background reading to traverse the map of your own body and draw out the mystery of your story, your body, your roots, your creativity and your life. You can begin with the rainbow warm-up and then work your way through each of the colours in the dance workshops, one by one. It is best to do this in sequence. You could spend at least a month on each colour, or even longer. In our training programme, we take two years to travel through the colours. Or you can start by doing one exploration week by week. As you read you will be drawn into the energy of each colour and chakra, so be aware of what is happening in your body, mind and emotions. You may have resistance to certain colours. If you find yourself resisting a colour then slow it down, take a break, come back to it later; you may be about to move through a major creative block. If one exploration doesn't suit you, then move to another. In our experience, great change can take place as people go through this alchemical journey and it is important to support yourself on every level as you move through the colours. For example, after one hour-and-a-half class in the colour red, one woman reported that she had gone home and slept right through the night for the first time in years. Another, who had been feeling sluggish and tired, said that she had felt so full of energy that she went home and cleaned her house from top to bottom. Two completely different results. Be aware of what is happening for you in each of the colours and note it down so you can use this knowledge when you need it. You can use the DTR process as a creative, healing and spiritual practice that will help you stay clear, grounded and focused. It will help you find more stillness in mind and emotions and you will be freer to dance to the rhythm of your own soul.

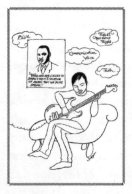

The Dance Workshops

Moving through the Spectrum

Exploring Red – Dancing our Roots: Chakra 1

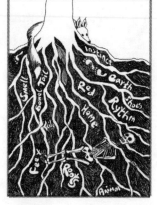

Key words or clues: roots, base of spine, feet, hands, sense of smell, skeletal and muscular system, movement downwards.

Base chakra	Root (Muladhara Sanskrit name)
Element	earth
Sense	smell
Affirmation	grounded – 'I *am* rooted in earth'
Colours	Red earthy colours, terracottas, clay, all the reds, e.g. vermillion, scarlet and dusty pinks
Location	base of spine, tail, anus, perineum, coccygeal plexus
Endocrine gland	related to the adrenals and the gonads, particularly the testes in the male
Secondary chakras	palms of the hands and soles of the feet

System	skeletal system, bones (marrow) associated with the muscular system
Clues	earth, roots, tail, grounding, sense of place, tribe, blood, home, body, bones, support, survival, fight/flight/freeze, stability, the basics, bowel, instinct, animal, rhythm, passion, courage
Symbols and props	bones, drums, rattles, earth, muck, shit, tribal images, body paint, skeleton/structure, branches, tail, feathers, fur, arrow pointing down, hut/house, shoes, money, land, ancestors, tribes, inheritance
Fragrance	ginger, patchouli, sage and, earthy scents
Food	root, root vegetables, red berries, red foods, mushrooms
Discipline	to be here *now* and to accept physical limitations; physically letting go; taking little steps to ground creative work; balance; grounding
Issues	bowel disorders, trouble with the legs and feet, e.g. varicose veins, piles; perfectionist/distaste of mess or unstructured time; fear of commitment or sticking with one thing, hopping from one thing to another; legs seem to have no energy; staying only with what feels safe; habitual behaviour, fear of change, movement, circulating; sluggish energy gathering around the buttocks and thighs; inability to stay grounded and in rhythm; suppressed anger, angry outbursts ('I saw red'); early suppressed trauma and abuse

Our feet plant themselves firmly on the ground.
We find or do not find support
We drop and tumble
And ever start again.

Raden Ayou Jodjana, *A book of self re-education*

Most of the writing in dancing with the instinctual body has been about grounding, support and healing the physical body and our roots, our family system, our ancestral heritage and the influence of our culture and landscape. This part of the work is where we begin to explore the dance and find ways to do this practically. Remember, in this first chakra we are connecting with the animal body – instinct – the skeletal system and our sense of smell. The associated parts of the body are: the root at the base of the spine – the tail, and the buttocks with the secondary chakras in the hands and feet.

These clues or attributes are the skeleton or bare bones of the work and, like the skeleton, they give structure and form to the dance. In order to ground our creativity in the world of form, we need a structure. Some structures become so big and unwieldy that energy coming through is stultified by the very thing that was supposed to help it. So we keep the structure light and easy, like a natural building that can be changed around and restructured if the energy coming in requires it. Grounding is the big clue here and we will explore what it means to ground in the dance and in our lives.

Some other clues we have are rhythm, home, freeze, fight or flight. We hone in on some of these clues directly and use others more subtly; for example, the sense of smell, by using incense, oils and fruits and releasing the scent into the room. Like a detective or an explorer, you are using these clues to explore the landscape of your own body. Each clue is there to guide you on your own creative journey. If we are not rooted or grounded, we cannot manifest our inspiration or creative dreams. By rooting I accept the limitation of the physical body and realise that there is only so much that I can practically ground in one lifetime or on any given day, therefore, I choose to follow my soul's priorities. We can acknowledge our own disabilities, physical trauma or hurt to the body and also the gifts and knowledge that come to us from our ancestors, our roots and the way we have learned to survive, heal and create. We can hold ourselves gently and allow ourselves to work at our own pace, following an inner rhythm in a gentle, playful way and with great respect for the wisdom of the body.

The Colour of Sound – suggested music for dancing your roots

·   African drum music / percussion is good and to begin we often use the slow rhythmic songs: from African artists, Baba Mal or Ayub Ogada, 'Obiero' from *En Mana Kuoyo*
·   Irish rhythmic music: *bodhrán* /drums, percussion. Artist Tommy Hayes, *A Room in the North*.
    Email agarvey@indigo.ie Ireland or perfgrp@aol.com
    Groups: Planxty Live 2004 and The Chieftans, for rhythm, storytelling, pacing.
    Kila, for wild exhuberance and breaking free.
·   *Rabhlaí Rabhlaí*: album of traditional rhymes with beautiful rhythms in Irish for children, with accompanying music. Good for children and adults. Editor, Roibeard O'Cathasaigh, Aoinad Forbartha Curaclain, Colaiste Mhuire, Gan Smal, Oll Scoil Luimnigh. Available at ansiopaleabhar@eircom.net
·   Aboriginal didgeridoo music for deep, resonant, communing with the roots
    Australian groups, Baka Beyond, *Spirit of the Forest*, Martin Cradick and Su White with the Baka Pygmies (good music for catharsis and deep shamanic communion with the body).
·   The music of Glen Velez, e.g. the album *Breathing Rhythms*. Good for connecting to heart beat, breath, and inner rhythms.
    Dreamland: *World Lullabies and Soothing Song*, Putumayo World Music

You can research your own earth music on the internet or in world music shops. Putumayo do a selection of some good music from different cultures. We would suggest that you go for the natural, simple, original music from the purest and most natural sources, mouth music, whistling, spoons, rattles, drums, didgeridoo. Try also to make your own rhythms with drums, hands on bodies, *bodhrán*, etc. Simple and slow is the key here. It does not have to be fast and impressive. Rhythms, sounds and rhymes to tune into your natural rhythms.

The Colour Red

When we are dancing the root chakra we use a variety of earthy colours that suit the group process and balance these with some of the cooler, complementary colours. By doing this we are clearing the murkier shades from the base chakra, and indeed the whole system, in a balanced and grounded way. This encourages the fresh, clear reds and pinks to flow down and through the roots. We are also clearing and cleaning these roots so that they can draw up fresh sap from the earth. Choose the colours that you are resonating with when you dance and trust your instinct on this.

The colour red is a great energiser and a good colour to treat anaemia. When the red ray is introduced into the system, it forms ions. These are minute particles that carry electro-magnetic energy in the physical body and affect the ferrous cell salt crystals, splitting them into iron and salt. The iron is absorbed and the salt is released through excretion. When the root is stimulated it causes adrenalin to be released into the blood stream. Red raises body temperature and improves circulation. It should not be used for people with high blood pressure or conditions like heart disease, as it is too powerful as a stimulant; use soft pink or coral instead in this case. Also, the cooler colours green and turquoise are especially good for blood pressure. In colour therapy we rarely use red on its own as it is too strong, or it can bring up strong emotions. However, it is fine to dance the base as this will help to balance and ground you. Indeed people on our courses often uncover long-standing blood pressure problems so that these can be dealt with before they become chronic. You can work with green or coloured flowers and plants to symbolise the roots. You can work with the earthy colours; dusty pink, terracotta, sandstone, or the clay reds and ochres. If you find these colours too strong, then use rose and different shades of pink. Poppy red is a lovely colour to use if you are suffering from inertia, or clay reds. Red flowers have their own integrity and you can balance the colour with lighter, cooler colours, for example, blue or turquoise.

In colour therapy where we are using coloured light as a healing tool, red's complementary colour is blue. This cool colour is good to use if you are raging or feeling violent or just too hot and burning in your body or if your blood pressure is high. Red energises and increases blood circulation, whereas the turquoise helps with any inflammations. Turquoise is very good for burns, or any burning infections, particularly throat infections. You can drape yourself with some silk scarves or place coloured bottles or candles around your house where you will see them every day. Or simply sit quietly and breathe in these colours.

By dancing the roots, you are beginning to build a relationship with the colour red in all its many shades. You can work with paint by adding black gradually to red paint. Then working with fresh red paint you can gradually add white. In this way you will get another sense of the colour and all the different shades. Notice how some reds are warm and others cooler because blue has been added. Mix red and violet and you will get shades of magenta, a very powerful colour which is helpful if you are teaching, organising or grounding creative work.

As you begin to build your relationship with the colours and in particular the earthier colours, you get to know them and become sensitive to their different nuances. Breathe the colours in, notice the different shades in nature. Let the mystery of the colour vibration move into your aura. Cut out different reds and earthy colours from magazines and stick them on a strip of cardboard. You can also combine colours using paint or tactile fabrics, until you find a combination that speaks to you. Eleanor has created a symphony of colour by creating a garden. Kate describes the newly nurtured green field of her garden as a canvas. This is intuitive work and very satisfying. You can also combine colours in the clothes you are wearing, a combination of different shades until you feel your body 'come alive'. One day your face might light up when you wear indigo and turquoise, another day this won't feel right and your body might need a soft pink or coral. When you see someone wearing the colours they are truly resonating with, and when they are moving in a grounded rhythmic way, the effect is startling. Like exotic birds of paradise they seem to come from a natural, vital planet, full of juicy, zestful energy.

Contemplate the colours by simply watching sunlight come through red glass. For example: look at the red in the stained glass windows in churches. Eventually we become more sensitive to colour and we know which shades will nurture and heal us in our clothes, in our environment and in the food we eat. There are many scientists now finding that red foods, for instance, have an affect on disease in the body. Think of bright orange carrot juice and green cabbage. These foods all bring their own healing vibration and colour is the key to the vibration they are bringing into the body. The colour of organic vegetables and flowers is so vibrant one can almost taste it just by looking. New discoveries tell us that organic foods have a higher capacity to store light than frozen foods, or foods that have been treated. The more light we receive from the sun and through our food and the elements, the healthier and more light filled we become. When we are attuned with nature we do not need experts to tell us this. We can sense it. Unfortunately with a lot of foods such as farmed salmon, the colours are added in a dye, not the same thing at all.

Breathe in the colours. Use your intuition to pick shades that you resonate with. You breathe the warming colours red, orange and yellow into your body through your feet. The green ray, which is the balance between the warm colours and the cooler colours, is breathed in horizontally through the heart centre. Blue, turquoise, indigo, violet, silver and gold are breathed in through the crown of the head. Breathe these colours into diseased parts of the body or into places where there is a stuck sensation, discomfort or pain. Trust yourself; if you breathe in a particular colour and then find that you don't want to breathe in that colour any more, trust that you have already done enough and your body is telling you to stop. It takes time for the body to integrate and digest these colours. We are sensitive instruments.

People who are angry need to avoid wearing red, but they certainly need to dance it. Really bright red is not good in kitchens where it is already hot, but can be lovely in big rooms that need warmth when used sparingly. Scarlet and gold are very powerful in a large room, but in smaller rooms use it in cushions, candles or curtains. Or use terracotta and gold. Be careful with dark reds or dirty reds, except when expressing emotionally with paint, unless you are using natural earth pigments which have their own integrity. For interior decorating, keep the colour clear, light and use sparingly. When using colour in your home refer to the light and how it will change the colours. I mix natural paint from limewash and natural pigments. The limewash reflects the light and the colours are not flat as they reflect nature in their shading like naturally dyed silk or cotton. It is soothing to watch the dappled light coming through the windows and turning the gold limewash into so many different hues. When the day is dull it changes again, and when it is damp the limewash absorbs the moisture from the air so that it darkens slightly, in this way changing with nature. It is the same with the body and the colours emanating from the body. When we work with the natural life force so close to nature, our colours are multifaceted, streaming and forever changing.

Artificial colours, chemicals, cleaners, medicines, perfumes, fabrics, etc. interfere with this natural dance. The effect is immediate and over time these have a deadening effect on the whole system, eventually leading to low energy and/or illness. People begin to look like whatever they are putting into and on their bodies. Artificial and man-made colours cannot compete with those created by nature.

As much as possible in the colours you use in your home, let them reflect nature; earthier colours on the floor, sky colours on the ceiling and greens in plants, cushions, walls, to bring a sense of balance. Also colours that reflect the day, relaxing blues and pinks in bedrooms, reflect the sunset and the approaching night but not indigo as it can cause nightmares. Also, if you are using violet you need to be working creatively yourself or it can cause depression. The brighter golds, oranges, greens and yellows are great in day places where we need energy to work. Even with very little money we can make paint or hang fabric, collect flowers and buy a candle so that the place we live is feeding us on every level. There are also coloured lights available now and natural light bulbs.

Remember that every colour has its complementary colour and sometimes small children see red as blue. If someone is wearing red, the blue ray is often seen around them. In the Steiner/ Waldorf schools, there is great knowledge about the effects of colour on the children and the colours are changed in the classroom to suit the children's developmental and creative process. So when you are dancing your roots it is important to nurture yourself on every level with good food, juices, beautiful colours, massage, oils and time spent in nature. You may also find that you need other support so that your body can be truly well.

Exploration: Body parts

- Bring your awareness down, down, down into the tail and the base of the spine.
- Open out the legs. Relax the shoulders; picture your tail as very long and balancing you.
- Let a sound into your throat, a low growl, coming up from the tail. Open and close your jaw and bare your teeth.
- Flex your hands and feet.
- Put the palms of your hands down towards the earth. Bend and soften your knees. Move your hands and feet, begin to wiggle your bottom and let that wiggle get right through your whole body, right through your spine.

- Put on some drumming music and explore some movement. Lead with your tail, the palms of your hands and
  the soles of your feet.

Let all your movements be soft, easy and effortless.

Exploration: Collage

- Explore your relationship with your tribe, the earth and
  your base chakra by making a collage.
- Use old magazines (*National Geographic* is good) – cut out
  pictures, images, words or colours and stick them on to a
  large piece of coloured card. You can add feathers, wool,
  string, coloured fabrics, shells, beads, whatever inspires you
  to create a tactile piece that you would like to touch.
- Hang this in your bedroom where you will see it every
  morning. Over time these images may begin creatively to
  communicate with you. You may be inspired to explore an
  animal you chose, either by painting or reading or simply
  dancing as that animal. Or you may want to explore your
  connection with a particular tribe, place or plant.
- Be aware of your dreams and write them out in the morn-
  ings as these archetypal images may begin to communicate with you through colour or through the animals and
  plants.
- Even if none of this happens, simply looking at these
  grounding images every morning will help you to come
  away from distressful or circular thinking and feel more
  connected with your body and the natural world.

You could also make a collage of your fears or the tribal fears of your
family and another collage of your own aspirations for your life.

Exploration: Walking Meditation

- Be mindful when you are walking.
- Open your legs more, use the soles of your feet and deliberately place the different areas of the sole of your foot onto the ground, e.g. from the heel to the ball of the foot, or try putting the ball of your foot down first and then the heel. Be mindful that you are treading the earth. The Native Americans say we are walking on the bones of our ancestors.
- Notice: Do you move close to the ground or bounce up and down? Do you come down heavily on your feet? Do you push your head forward or look up at the sky.
- Put on some African drum music and walk with an awareness of your bones, your skeleton.
- Connect to earth, heartbeat and breath.
- Practise staying with your heart and breath rhythm, notice when you push against it or fight it.
- Be aware of your thoughts and how they can stiffen up your body as if they have to keep it upright. Let your body hold itself up.
- Notice the way you place your feet on the ground and let your eyes take in your surroundings.
- Listen to the birds and your breath. Notice the different rhythms and sounds within your own body and in the landscape around you.
- Imitate other people's walks. How does it feel to walk like a cool dude or a model who may be pointing toes inwards and stiffening the hips?
- When you are walking, notice when you cut off your breath or rise up from the ground.
- After you have walked, lie still on the earth and feel it holding every part of your body – every cell, every breath. Breathe with the earth.

Exploration: Dancing the Bones 1

Having worked with rhythm for many years Antoinette says, 'rhythm is a whole universe of instinctive knowledge and ways of being. Africa is the place on this earth whose traditions contain some of the most sophisticated knowledge of rhythm patterns and their conscious use in generating different states of being or invoking different energies.' Let's explore this now in our own bodies by dancing the bones.

- Close your eyes and see if you can scan the skeleton of your body with your inner awareness.
- You do not need to know the names of the bones, simply sense into your bones.
- When we see pictures of skeletons, they are usually uniform skeletons, however, everyone's bones are different – all different shapes with unexpected curves in the spine or perhaps one shoulder is higher than the other or a right hip is higher than a left. Each skeleton is unique – the shape and weight of the bones and the way that skeleton stands in space.
- See your skeleton as a tree that has been shaped by the winds and the landscape in which it has grown.
- Notice where your pelvis is and your shoulders above your pelvis. Where is your head? How are all of these balancing? Where are your legs and your feet? What shape does your skeleton make in the space?
- Try out a few different shapes or pictures, leading with your elbow first. Then the shoulder joint. Then a knee. You are creating different sculptured shapes with your bones and muscles.
- Extend your arm and push into the wrist, release slowly. Push into the fingers, release slowly. Push into your hip bone and release slowly. Travel through your body like this, pushing into a bone or joint and releasing. Push – breathe in, release – breathe out.
- Feel the solidity of the bones and the weight of them. Some are heavy and long, others quite fragile and light.

- Begin to find your own rhythm now, tuning into the different weights and sensations in your bones and muscles.
- Working without music, find your own rhythm and sense of timing as you dance your bones. Sense into the rhythm of these bones clacking together, the echo down through the body and the beat of your heart and blood pulsing through your body.

Exploration: Dancing the Bones 2 (Deirdre's dance)

Deirdre O'Connor, one of our trainers, led us all in the bone dance. She found a good rhythmic piece of drum music, not too fast and not too slow. Then we began by dancing the bones from the toes upwards. This is a good rhythmic, lively dance and the bones come alive when you focus your attention on them and ask them to communicate to each other in this way.

- Move and dance the small bones in your toes, then extend to all the bones in your feet
- Ankle joints then lower leg
- Dance your knees, then thighs and so on
- Travel up through the body, thigh bones, hip bones, pelvis, lower spine; take your time. Dance the vertebrae, then the ribs, collar bones, shoulder blades, upper spine, neck, cranial bones, the bones in your face, fingers, hands, wrists, elbows, upper arms and so on until all your bones are dancing from the inside out

Exploration: Connecting with your Inner Rhythms

- Focus on your heartbeat and breath and the pulse of your blood moving through your body.
- During the day, practise staying with your own rhythm; notice when you push against it or fight it.
- Notice when you try to beat the clock; what happens to your breath?

- Notice the way you stiffen your body as if your mind has to keep it upright. Practise letting go with your mind and letting your body's natural rhythm take over.
- Keep your working rhythm steady.
- Keep coming back from the tendency to speed up and go out of rhythm. Notice when you are engaged in one task and you begin to think of something else you should or could be doing. What happens to your body and breath?
- If your head is too full of thoughts and you are experiencing anxiety or are overwhelmed, stamp like a two year old; bring all the notions down from your head and let them go into the earth. Keep the rhythm as you stamp.
- Walk. Skip. Hop. Jump. Stamp.
- Beat out little rhythms on the car dashboard or on your body or any surface near to you. Two people could play a rhythm massage game on each others bodies.
- When lying in the bath, you can get your circulation moving by cupping your hands and drumming on the different parts of your body. This is great on the thighs. Notice the different echoes and sounds on different parts of your flesh. Add in clapping and clicking.
- Listen to drumming or other rhythmic music. Let the bones of your body connect with the drum beat.
- Attune your body to the rhythms in nature by noticing patterns birds make in the sky, the rhythmic movement of the wings, the way the different songbirds use different rhythms. Listen to a purring cat or a barking dog.
- Notice music being played in cafés or shops and the effect it is having on you. Notice if it is pulling you away from your own sense of rhythm or echoing it.
- Become aware of your inner rhythms. If possible, on a day off, take time to follow this inner rhythm. Trust it. If you don't get up until one, then trust that. Perhaps you feel like breakfast at three o'clock or in the middle of the night; trust that as well. Try to listen to your own body, not what experts are telling you. You are listening below the habitual addictive tendencies

that you use to get through a day where you might be pushing yourself. For example, if you are automatically reaching for the chocolate, ask yourself – is this what you really want or are you taking it because you need to sleep? Then you may decide no, I really want this, but check that it isn't an automatic, habitual thing.

- When you are on holidays, take each day at a time and see if you can begin to live to a rhythm that arises from within rather than one imposed by the world's schedules, or your surface 'should do's'.
- Try this now for a moment: close your eyes, breathe, be free for just a moment, let your hands touch your body or rise up over your head. Set your body free of the constraints of your thoughts. Listen to the sounds in nature or the sounds around you. Gaze around you without locking your eyes on any one thing. Breathe.
- Say, 'I am free, I am free to follow my own inner rhythm, my sense of timing is accurate; my body knows how to be.'
- Listen to your breath, take your pulse; if possible do this outside and connect with the rain, the currents of air, the birdsong and your bare feet on the ground.

Exploration: Singing the Bones

This is a wonderful way to commune with your body in a way that it understands.

- Begin by connecting with your bones.
- Start humming to your bones, start intuitively with the bones of your feet or your ankles or your fingers, and then allow the bones to hum back to you. When you get good at this, you can connect with deeper bones like the bones of your pelvis. You can even connect with one vertebra at a time.
- Take time afterwards to sit with your bones and then let your bones write or paint to you.

- When you have practised this, you could bring a tape machine and tape these songs and maybe add some words.

Exploration: Your Earthy Man or Woman

- Can you think of someone who to you is an earthy man or woman? This symbolic person can help you to ground if you are feeling anxious.
- Practise walking with your legs open and your feet trudging into the earth like an old farmer walking his land, each step a punctuation.
- Take time to sense the rhythm of this walk. Notice your pace and the way you might drop your hips and your whole body, your jaw, your shoulders down towards the earth.
- Walk in places where people have always walked; holy places, old places. Even built-up areas have a history in the land; find out what it is.
- Make your own pilgrimages. If you are confused in your life and do not know what direction to take, then take the time to walk somewhere, or travel to a holy place or a place that has always resonated with you. Even if you cannot actually go there, you can go to the river or the well or simply sit with a bowl of earth and connect with that distant place. Ask the land to guide you, particularly when you are in those places that seem to have a magical, fairy feel about them – a little tree grove, or bushes near a stream or river, fairy raths covered in old trees or a stone circle.
- Spend time with a particular plant or flower.
- Notice how nature's wilderness steals through the concrete, finds roots in unexpected places. Notice how nature is always there.

Exploration: The Homeplace

- In the early years of your life, where did you live?
- Were you born in a hospital or at home?
- What was the local accent like?
- Find pictures of the houses you lived in. Did you move house a lot?
- Were you ever homeless?
- Were you abandoned?
- What do you love about certain places?
- Can you gather stones, shells, wood or clay from these places or a local song, story or book?
- What sort of clan are you from? What way did they move, stand and what did they wear? What were their survival issues? What way did they fight?
- If you were making a film about your clan, what sort of props would you use? For example, if I were to make a mythical film or play about one of my family homes I would fill one room with old top hats, canes, costumes, tap shoes and another with bills, certain books, photographs and the waste-disposal units and microwaves and pieces of kitchens and other gadgets that my father was selling at that time. I would also have a long dark corridor with a door at the end of it and the sound of my mother singing old Broadway songs with a Dublin accent, and occasionally I would have pigeons flying over the occupants to catch my fathers childhood memories of rearing pigeons and also his erratic genius as he had these flights of fancy that took him into new creative ventures while abandoning the old ones.
- If you were going to make a film about your clan of origin, who would you cast to play your mother, your father, your sister, brother, yourself and so on? Why are you picking these particular actors? What qualities do they have that resonate with the qualities within your clan of origin? If you cannot bear to do this, then create a new cast and clan with the qualities you would have liked in your life or would like to bring into your life now.

- Write a short story, or a poem or make a collage about a scene from your life. Stand back and look at the people as if they were characters from a novel or a film. Use your imagination. It could be a detective novel, a romance, science fiction or it could be about a dark anti-hero. Hone in on key phrases, the way people move and act, the way they look when they are trying to hide something. Obviously, only work with what you feel able for.
- Who are your tribe now? Who do you hang out with?
- What makes you feel at home? The smell of cooking or freshly baked bread? A real fire? A candle? A storybook? A big blanket?
- Explore what makes you feel at home and see if it links with old memories of home or even of a friend's home or describe a safe home where you would like to live. You can go to this safe place within your own body when you feel anxious or afraid.

Practise walking like your earthy man or woman, see if you can embody the qualities you are sensing in them through your dance.

Exploration: Oiling the Joints

- Stiffen your joints and then release them. As you stiffen them, notice what happens to the rest of your body. See if you can breathe even as you contract.
- Practise walking around with stiff joints and a stiff expression on your face, as if you were a robot with mechanical joints and limbs.
- Be aware that energy often gets stuck in the joints. To help to release this, you can move your joints slowly while breathing a pale watery pink into the joints, or whatever colour comes to you intuitively.
- Practise walking with your shoulders and hips moving. Let your arms and legs be loose, especially at the joints.

- Throw out your legs and arms in a loose, disjointed fashion.
- Let your body flop about like a rag doll.
- Leave your jaw loose and let spontaneous sounds come as you flop around.
- Extend your arms and then slowly release from the joints. First fingers, then wrists, elbows, shoulders. Keep checking that you are not holding your breath.
- Now do the same with your legs. Hold onto something, extend one leg backwards. Hold the tension in your muscles and joints and use your voice to groan and sound as you do this.
- Then slowly release your leg from the toes right up to the hip, while breathing and making gentle little groaning sounds.
- Walk around and notice the difference in the two legs before extending the other leg.
- Move the joints on one side of the body and then compare them to the other side.
- Massage one foot thoroughly and then compare it to the other.
- You can also release and harmonise stuck energy by using your voice. Breathe in the colour and then send your voice down into your body, letting it massage these stiff places. Your voice can move into all those hidden tendons and ligaments and give expression to the aches or stiffness there.

Exploration: Animal Meditation

You can tape this meditation or read it first then go through the steps.

- Lie down and close your eyes.
- You are an animal, warm and safe, lying underground in your lair.

- You have a big jaw and sharp teeth. Paws with claws. A strong intelligent sense of smell. You have thick fur on your back and soft fur on your belly.
- Are there other animals lying close beside you? You can snuffle up against them. You are making soft, guttural sounds and move your body in a sensual way as you burrow more deeply into the earth and rest.
- Listen to the sounds around you and notice the smells. Your sense of smell travels right through your body down through the spine and tail.
- When you move your tail, your whole spine tingles right up to your ears.
- Although you are resting deeply, you are fully alert and ready to spring into action, your strong haunches propelling you forward, the wide sweep of your belly revealed as you leap in the air using your springy spine.
- As you lie there, sense what it would be like for you to run close to the earth and the distance you can cover, to leap up high, to crouch low; to move through your territory that is absolutely familiar and has your smell on it.
- Sense what it is like to be able to find your own food to hunt and kill and to tear at the flesh with your big wide jaw. You can scratch with your paws and tear at the undergrowth.
- All the time you are sensing the other animals, those that you ignore, those that are prey and those that prey upon you.
- You are wild and strong and the wildness around you is a part of you.
- Now breathe deeply into your animal body and prepare to move, languidly at first.
- You can move as the animal or hold the spirit of the animal in your body as you dance.
- Sniff out the room you are in and the nature all around you; move instinctively through the place.
- Find the warm places to lie or crawl; move close to the

bodies you want to be beside. You have no need to be polite. You can sniff at other bodies and then move away. Above all else you are following your instincts.

· Gently come out of the meditation, but thank the animal in you and ask this animal to work with you. It does not have to be any particular animal; simply get a sense of the animal body and the wild earthy smell along with the instinctive natural way of mating, hunting, eating, defecating and fighting.

Let this body knowledge inform your movements and way of being. Practise in your life as you walk down a street or as you enter a room, reconnect with this instinctive way of moving and being. Slow didgedridoo music is good for this.

Exploration: The Squat

· The squat is a very powerful position to ground and root your body and your creative dreams.

· Yoga squats are very helpful. If you don't do yoga, then simply squat down using your hands to balance you or you can hang onto a low table or rail.

· See if you can put your feet flat on the ground. If not, stay on the balls of your feet but gradually over time let your feet flatten out.

· It can be helpful to find opportunities to squat down, for example on the phone, or sorting things on the floor. If we had not been taught to sit in chairs, we would do this quite naturally as a small child does with posture beautiful to observe.

· Begin to observe the whole process of defecation and you may begin to notice more subtle effects. It's valuable learning about energy, fear and instinct.

· Notice what parts of you are stiffening up and where you are relaxed and at ease.

· When you get comfortable in the squat, try groaning from

the base of the body. Be careful not to make the sound from your neck. Relax your jaw and throat: now begin to make a deep didgeridoo sound. This groaning allows the lower body to open out and relax and is very helpful for women in labour or for any birthing process and also for releasing stagnant energy and grounding the body.

This exploration is also useful to people who may be suffering from irritable bowel syndrome, constipation or other disorders as it allows the pelvis to open out and the lower body to re-align properly supporting the internal organs and the whole process of elimination.

Exploration: Study Animals

· Training a cat to use a cat tray in the house, I watched the efficient way she used her whole body to defecate. The paws and legs, the spine and belly. Look at animals and see how graceful and natural they are in all their movements

· Look at wildlife programmes and imitate the movements of the animals. What does that feel like in my body? Of course, television does not provide the authentic smells my cat so kindly bestowed on me, immediately teaching me how the sense of smell is connected with the root.

Exploration: Make a Tail

· Gather materials and see if you can make a tail. You could use twine, fur or any other old materials like beads and wool.

· You can attach the tail onto you and shake and wave it when you dance or you can hang it on your wall as a symbolic grounding image that will remind you to detach from your thoughts and bring your awareness down into your physical body.

Exploration: Connecting with your Roots

- The energy in the base is downwards and outwards. The roots pushing down with the sap rising. Get a sense of this in your body. The more you connect with the earth, the more the sap can rise. When we contract and hold back from that pushing in the tail, legs and feet, particularly in the joints, we disconnect and the sap cannot rise.

- Practise pushing against something; for example, a bean bag against a wall. Be like a baby animal pushing its way out of the womb.

- Push with your feet and push with the palms of your hands. Let the movements be sensual, but use your energy to push. Let your body writhe and slither, like a snake.

- Bring your jaw into it and your voice. Grunting and groaning. Let your spine curl.

- Explore this for yourself. It may begin to feel very satisfying. Bring in cat movements, curving your spine and then arching your back.

- Stretch out completely, pushing upwards with your hands and downwards with your feet very slowly. Allow the muscles to gradually let go of the stretch, notice how that feels in every fibre of your body.

- Then repeat: let your spine extend and open your mouth, then once again slowly let the muscles relax. The energy really begins to shift in the very slow relaxation of the muscles after the stretch. If at any time your body shakes, let that shaking move through the muscles or use that shaking to make a sound if that feels comfortable for you.

Exploration: Body Release

- If your body needs to release old, stuck or unbalanced energy, pick music or work in silence, and begin to follow the movements in your body.

- Check if this feels safe. If not, work with a movement or body worker.

- If it feels safe in your body, dance and let your body lead. Your body may tremble or make unexpected movements. You may move vigorously or gently. Then you might want to lie very still – let this happen as best you can without thoughts and emotions interfering, but stay present to the sensations in your body. Don't abandon yourself and don't over-dramatise with strong emotions, let the body do it.
- If you begin to experience strong emotions, come gently back. All the time you are moving be aware of your thoughts and emotions, but go just below them to the sensation in your body. For example: I feel heat around my heart, my throat feels tight, or my feet are hot and itchy and my mouth is turning down or my stomach feels squishy; I want to twist my body, and when I do I can feel a little tremor in my shoulder. Staying with the body sensations keeps you safe and grounded. If you cannot find words to describe the sensations in your body, use sounds. My nose feels all 'mnghee'. I feel my nervous system going 'eeeeeeeee'.
- If you find your thoughts are speeding up or you feel afraid, stop, breathe and walk around. Do not force or push yourself in any way. If you feel impatience or anger with yourself, be careful not to let that anger push you. If you find that you are doing that, find someone to work with you. The impatience often wants a quick answer or a quick solution, and is a way of avoiding the natural healing that needs to take place in the body first, only later will the thoughts catch up.
- You can express anger in a dance so that it does not bully the child within. See the child within as being wrapped and protected in a pink light.
- I often shook, danced and then slept for a half an hour. The instinctual intelligence in the body knows how to heal itself, if you give it the time and space.
- Have some paint or crayons to hand. Don't try and make

an image, work with the colours. Use your hands and feet and allow yourself to make a mess.

· Put your paintings and colours on your altar.

Exploration: Identify your Pattern of Tensing

· Can you identify your pattern of tensing? Jaw, face, arms, legs, knees, feet, tummy, bottom, hips, shoulders, neck. Also the inner body: the gut, the bowel and so on. Begin to observe when and how you are tensing up.

· Where is your body most tense?

· Where in your body are you most relaxed, free and light?

· What parts of your body can you breathe into? Where does the breath stop?

· Where do you experience numbness or a kind of plastic body sensation?

· Where in the body are you feeling sensation, even pain?

· Notice, without judgement, habitual body gestures and postures.

Play some gentle, safe music and begin to make a small dance, calling on these different sensations, gestures and postures to inform your movements.

Exploration: Moving through Rage and into Passion
Warm up first.

· If you have rage that can be felt in the tail, wave it like a cat and let your hackles rise, slowly explore it through movement. Growl, use your hands to scratch and maul like a tiger. Open your jaw and let out the sound. Hit out if you want, but keep it loose and keep a rhythm going.

· Check if the body is really angry; sometimes we might think we are ready to fight and find that the body wants to do a gentle easy dance or hum a soothing tune.

- Sometimes we really need to explore suppressed energy. SLOW IT RIGHT DOWN: Notice your breath and how you might hold it or try to control the energy. Notice where strong energy or sensation is in your body. Notice where you are holding onto it. Notice if you are lifting up out of your body. Notice if your thoughts are becoming impatient and wanting to 'Get it out'. Don't try to 'Get it out'.
- Sense into your own process and how your body has coped up to now. Be gentle. Do not go with the strong momentum of it. Slow it down.
- See if you can sound your anger. Does the sound connect with the root of it? If not, where does it disconnect or where is it missing?
- Don't waste your time putting your anger on other people by going into your thoughts to see where it belongs. Stay with the sensation of it curling through your own body.
- Keep connecting with your throat, tail, belly and jaw. If your body contracts, go with that contracting.
- Let the rage rise physically like a wave coming up from the feet and then ground it back down through the body and into the feet.
- Stay with it for as long as it feels safe. Simply follow your body and see where it leads.
- You are simply staying with something that has been going on for years, but now you are allowing the animal body to be with it. Like a dammed river, the energy will find a way through without you controlling it.
- Relax, make a game of it, even with the distress and pain we all experience, the animal body is still fascinating, particularly when we can connect with the clean impulses of that body below the surface thoughts. Work with support when possible, but you are the one who does the work.
- Dance to the drum: it creeps up the legs, and whoa, volcano time, keep the rhythm but let it surge, body moving to it, pulsing with it. Warrior dance. Passionate flamenco. Move from one foot to another, push into your heel, into

the ball of your foot, loosen out the base of your spine.

- All that power, all that courage, not to use against anyone else, but to use when rat voices begin to scuttle in the attic whispering their venomous put-downs and fear does its ghostly dance. Stay with it, feel it in your body, use it in your dance, own it, use it and then let it go.

- When you are dancing, you may feel a heavy tiredness coming on; slow the movements, pace yourself and breathe more deeply. Connect with the drums, then the energy can surge up from the earth; a fresh new energy that flows upwards through your body and throws off the debilitating tiredness.

NB If your rage feels out of control or overwhelming, do the work with a support person. Also, if you feel the need to hit something with a stick, be careful how you do this. Do a warm-up first, then position yourself firmly on your feet, keep your knees soft and make sure your spine and neck are flexible, then raise your arms and shoulders, use your whole body and breath. As you hit the object, expel your breath and make a sound if you can. Stay connected in the base and don't allow the anger to hurt you. I often see people hitting things but they are not breathing and they are restricted around the shoulders and upper arms so even though there is some movement of energy it still appears impotent. It is most important to feel the energy pumping freely through a flexible body. Be careful not to stiffen up your jaw and neck. You can snarl and let the sound come from deep inside. Be careful of your voice and larynx, you only need to do this a few times so you can feel the energy moving; otherwise it becomes habitual. Then you can move on by making a warrior dance by using a stick or sword. Afterwards you could make sounds, write or paint.

Exploration: Predator/Prey
- If you are feeling fearful, choose an animal, e.g. a rabbit, to represent that fear.
- Ask this animal to help you with your fear.
- Let the sensation of being this animal come into your body. Wait until you feel the impulse to move before you begin your dance. Don't try to look like or dance like a rabbit, allow your body to express the rabbit in its own way.
- Notice how your body feels and expresses itself.
- When you feel complete, breathe, stretch and relax, then thank your animal for helping you.
- When you are ready, choose an animal that would represent the predator for you then follow the exploration as you did before, again coming to completion.
- Now see if you can bring these two animals together in your body. Perhaps they live in two different chakras. Move to the energy of one animal and then another. Now create a dance combining the two energies.

Make the dance as seamless as possible, letting your movements from one animal flow into another so that if there were people watching they would be unaware that these were two separate dances.

Exploration: Instinctual Intelligence
- Practise following the instinctual intelligence in your body. Start with a minute or two, then five minutes and then fifteen and so on.
- You can do this by first of all becoming aware of your thoughts and standing back a little from them, observing them but not caught up in them.
- Now notice your emotions, how you are feeling right now; afraid, sad, angry, excited, numb.
- Next notice the sensations in your body, places where you

are hot or cold or stiff or tense or wriggly, find your own words, or even better, sounds.
· Lastly notice any tingling in the body. Breathe and let yourself sink into this fine, pure sensation and notice the energy of it through your whole body, in some places light, other places deeper or denser.

Move now from this purified instinct, this intelligence that is faster than thought or emotion. Even if you simply move a finger or an eyelid, these movements are very precious and inform and fill your body and life with stillness. Movement and physical expression quietens the mind and emotions and so the inner world is still even if the body is moving. BREATHE.

Exploration: Sense of Smell and the Aura
· When you see a flower or plant that you love, take the time to stop and inhale the scent.
· Choose one of the flowers, or if it is something like gorse select some of the yellow flowers to focus on. Let your eyes be soft in their focus.
· Inhale the scent, gazing at the flower. Now close your eyes and see the flower in your mind's eye.
· Repeat this three times.
· You will notice that the essence of the flower travels subtly through your body.
· If you do this with a number of flowers the sensation in the body is erotic and deeply sensual as if the essence of the plants makes love to you and you to the plant.
· When you have communed closely with the flower, see yourself as a bird rising above the landscape, and notice where the plant is growing and what other plants are growing around it.
· Smell the landscape and the earth in that place.
· Notice the smells in your own house and place. Be conscious of the fragrance and the effect of fragrance on your

body or on other peoples' bodies when they enter your home.

- Keep the fragrances natural as synthetic fragrances have a synthetic effect on the body. Natural fragrances harmonise the energies in the body and in the home.
- You can also call a plant or flower to mind. See it in your mind's eye and inhale the smell. The essence of that plant or flower will come to you. This is plant medicine.
- Flower essences are wonderful ways to take in the healing power of the plant. Especially if you are feeling distracted and cannot settle to commune with nature. Flower essences heal on a subtle vibratory level because the flowers are so close to the source, the instinctual intelligence in all nature. When you inhale and take in the essence of a living, growing plant, you come closer to that essence within your own body.

EXPLORING ORANGE – FLUID DANCE: CHAKRA 2

Key words or clues: pelvic bowl, hips, wrists, ankles, body fluids, emotional body; movements are circular, moving inwards.

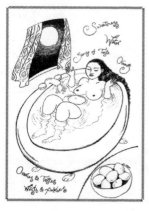

Main attributes

Sacral area	sweetness/swadhisthana (Sanskrit word)
Element	water
Sense	taste
Affirmation	permission to rest
Colours	orange, rich sensual colours, marigold, coral
Location	lower abdomen
Endocrine glands	ovaries and testes
Secondary chakras	wrists, ankles
System	reproductive system, lymphatic system
Clues	water, moon, female/yin, relationship, creativity, desire, seeds, intimacy, sweetness, sensuality, grooming, goddess; dark/black/emptiness, negating, receiving, sensation, reflecting, waiting, resting, syrupy, joy
Symbols and props	oval, egg, moon, wavy water lines, ancient symbols, containers, bowls, jugs, basket, shells, shawls, woven cloth, web, net, mermaid, goddess, dolls, cave, womb, dolphin, whale, snake, childhood images, orange flowers, pomegranate, river, lake, sea, seeds
Fragrance	rose, orange, neroli
Food	shellfish, oranges, orange foods, juice, seeds, eggs
Discipline	containment of sexual-emotional energy, tuning into and refining one's inner creative

	process, letting go of old emotional baggage, stillness
Issues	inability to rest, guilt, problems with the reproductive system, sexual and emotional abuse, enmeshment, seduction, blocks to intimacy/ creativity, manipulation dryness, rigidity, disrespect, bitterness, inability to give and receive

The other women are the same as ever.
No one has peeped into their inmost being,
and they themselves know not their own secret.

Rabindranath Tagore

As we prepare to enter the energy of this chakra, we begin by invoking the element water. We tune into our fluidity: the streams, rivers and seas of the body and this energy that spirals inwards. This is the sacral centre, the yin, female receptive energy, associated with the moon, the dark woman, goddess, fertility, joy, sweetness, sexuality and the juices of life. The colour orange with its complementary chakra colour indigo is represented by the image of the seed and the egg and of course, the chalice. These images give us the clues we need to explore this element within the body. When we dance we move our hips, the pelvic bowl and the secondary chakras by moving our ankles and wrists. Our movements are undulating, reflective, and sensual as we explore watery, fluid movements and the life-giving essence in this chakra.

Here we are working with the reproductive system and creativity, and also with the lymphatic system and fluids in the body.

We are fine-tuning and deepening our capacity to explore our emotions, our sensuality, our creativity and our ability to contain all of this within fluid boundaries as we connect with the stillness at the bottom of this well. Once again we can hone in on some of the clues (archetypes and associations) directly and use others more subtly. For example, we can explore the sense of taste by peeling oranges and feeding them to each other or practice present moment awareness and bring a meditative quality to the preparation and eating of food. This draws on our sensuality in many ways, like moving our tongues to taste the fluids in our mouths.

In this colour we connect with the purest form of the female essence. This essence is light and sweet and lies just below the turgid energy in the belly. We can get caught in the vortex of emotions that keep changing and leading us on a tiring dance and it is here we learn to contain and work with our emotions in a conscious way and to connect with the stillness that lies beneath. The unconscious becomes conscious but not in a linear way where it can be described in an academic thesis. It is in the bend of your back, the twist of your wrist and the wild song that rises unbidden from the belly.

Music

Listen for a watery, syrupy quality in your music or in the voice of the singer; a voice that slides through the scales and flows around the notes.

- Music by artists such as Deva Premal, Sheila Chandra, Loreena McKennit.
- Jai Uttal, *Footprints* – Don Cherry and Laksmi Shankar
- *Gipsy Music – the rough guide to the music of the gypsies* www. worldmusic.net / www.roughguides.com/music
- Theme music from the films *Monsoon Wedding*, Michael Danna and *Chocolat*, Rachel Portman (Sony Music)
- Traditional and new, folk and circle dance music.
- Flamenco, Jewish folk songs, Egyptian, Indian sacred music and song, some *sean-nós* singing, e.g. Liam Ó Maonlaí, Sinead O'Connor, Kíla, Losarina
- Water sounds, whale sounds.

Once again look for the sacred, fluid music that grounds and connects you to the deep belly. Some of this music can be more third eye and trancelike. You are looking for music that draws you down into the hips and belly. The music and dance can bring about an ecstatic state, but it is grounded and sensual.

The Colours around you – Orange

Bright orange in the aura shows zest, health and juiciness for life. The colour increases confidence and vitality. This colour is often connected with youth and joy and it energises the system. If you are tired, exhausted or shocked then use pale orange or peach. This orange ray is often used to treat kidney stones and gallstones. Orange is also used to treat ovarian cysts and for the reproductive system in general. It is good for fatigue and depression. It builds up our immune system and helps to break up mucus in the system, so it is very good for chest conditions and cloggy, stuck energy, particularly in the lymphatic system. The orange ray recharges the etheric body which connects the physical body to the life force coming into it. Use it with the complementary indigo for balance.

Paler oranges are relaxing and encourage us to be creative. Soft peaches are good colours to use in our homes and, if they suit us, in our clothes. Bright orange can bring up our emotions too quickly, so work firstly with peach and the bright orange in candles and flowers. Use blue for balance.

You can use neroli (orange flower-blossom) and orange essential oils in the oil burner. Neroli has a light, subtle perfume. Massage with neroli, jasmine or rose oil. The use of orange can bring on a desire to cook nourishing meals and create beauty in our homes and surroundings. As we nurture ourselves in this way, we will notice guilt giving way to pleasure and when food is prepared with love it satisfies us so we are not empty and hungry all the time.

This colour will also connect us with our sensuality and the juicy energy that lies within. It may also bring up any health issues that need to be looked after.

Exploration: The Fluid Body

This exploration is for tuning into the fluid body at different levels and bringing this fluidity into movement.

- Hips, pelvis, wrists and ankles; bring your awareness to these body parts in silence and contemplation.
- Sense the fluids moving through your body.
- Connect with the sense of taste, your mouth and tongue, the orange colour.
- Keep your legs soft, knees slightly bent. Let your body relax as if you were sinking into warm water.
- Move your legs and hips as if you were walking through water, hands trailing the waves.
- See water with the third eye: sea, lake, stream, river. Feel the different atmosphere of each one as you move. The still lake, a wild sea, a babbling brook, a deep flowing river. Let your movements reflect these different atmospheres.
- Settle into the water, rising on the in breath, sinking even lower on the out breath.
- Rise up to the surface and then sink down again.
- Lie on the floor and let your body be moved by the water, little movements at first then bigger, rising and sinking. Become the waves, become the still, deep flow of the river.
- Explore this fluid body and notice the difference in your body when you connect with the fluids in comparison to the bones and muscles.

Exploration: Golden Liquid

For reflection and centring – softens and relaxes the whole system.

- Begin to move this little thimble of golden fluid deep in your belly.
- Sense the movement, tiny, tiny not even reaching your outer body.
- Eyes are gazing inward; reflective, waiting. Tune into the subtlest sensations.
- Swirl this golden liquid in the thimble and then see this thimble grow bigger into a bowl and you can swirl your

hips so the liquid is swirling and you are being careful not to spill any of this precious fluid.

· Feel the syrupy sensations that trickle from the belly and emanate outwards, golden honey spreading through the fluids of the body.

· Remember that the bones and skeleton were formed in water, the waters of the womb, so allow the bones to float in this liquid.

· Move your hips in every direction, letting your body follow. Rotate your wrists and ankles.

· Stay grounded and keep your connection with your tail, feet and hands.

· Finish by breathing in this honey, golden colour and breathing it gently outwards through the pores of the skin.

Exploration: Create an Altar

· Gather the seeds to heal. Let them flow to you.
· Begin with an empty bowl or a bowl of water.
· See what colours or feminine symbols, music, poems or images come to you. In student workbooks we often see copies of the old paintings of women looking into water or bathing together, the woman raising her face out of the water to the man who is gazing down at her. Or we see images of women dancing with veils and bracelets on their wrists and ankles.
· Find images or objects that are meaningful for you. Play music while looking, touching and arranging them.

Exploration: The Female Way – To Explore the Inner Feminine

· As you move your hips and wrists, ask your inner female to help you to slow down and connect with her.
· Be conscious of the ways she communicates, in a song on the radio, the essence in a flower, a subtle fragrance or a

colour. She may be in a young girl's smile, a woman's hair, the strong, slow, deep voice of a man who has touched her essence. This is knowing that comes from the belly, a silky water movement.

· Let these images and sensations be seeds for your dances, songs and stories.

Exploration: Water Meets Earth

Becoming conscious of the interrelationship between the earth and the fluid body, exploring inner and outer movement.

· Dance the element earth and then move into the element water, noticing the transition from one element to another.
· This is an edge place: a meeting of water and earth; the waves on the sand or the cliff over the sea.
· We could jump or run and plunge. Hold our breath, push down and plunge, or take it gently. Feel the change of element and the caress of water on your skin.
· Let your fingers trail the water, sense the cold or heat of it. Splash with your hands then move quickly, then slowly with your hands through the water. Try bending and twisting your wrists and fingers and then your arms.
· Lower yourself slowly into a warm bath. Take time to notice how the water parts to receive you and how your body softens under the water's caress.
· Water does not travel in straight lines; it meanders and ripples. Let your movements mimic this.
· Go with the cycles in your belly. Become languorous as you slow down and walk along, gently moving your hips from side to side and sinking down into each hip as you walk.
· Connect with the waxing and waning moon. Notice the different quality of your movements and your rest.
· As you lie in water, notice how your bones feel and then your muscles.
· Before you enter a river or the sea, take time to introduce

yourself to the landscape there. Be aware of the mountains and the trees waiting there; be conscious of your entry into a place that they have lived for thousands and thousands of years.

· Ask for permission to enter the water and ask the water to help you to commune with the living landscape.

Exploration: Emptying the Vessel

It is important to clear away old desires and dreams that may be filling the space, dissipating the energy and not allowing current dreams to manifest. For example, one of our dancers wanted to be a nun when she was a child and also a mother with eight children! As a child, another dancer had wanted to be an actor and a singer and she found she was still looking at posters and wondering if she would ever go to drama college. She didn't really want to do that any more as she wanted to put energy into following her number one desire, but she noticed how distracted she was becoming with all these old desires still pulling on her.

· Make a list of all the dreams and aspirations you ever had.
· Become these roles in your body. Walk around as the person you might have become, make a dance out of it.
· Honour this creative part of you and after the dance let this part of you write and paint.
· Make a list of old lovers who you still think about or people you would have liked to have a relationship with
· Look at your lists, notice, is there a repeating theme that is moving through your life.
· Now clear and balance the sacral energy of these old dreams that may be out of date. Do this by seeing white fluid light moving through your body, clearing and balancing the energy there.
· You have now created an empty vessel and allowed the space for something fresh and new to unfold. It may have

connections with these old dreams that you have made more conscious, or it may be a whole new dream.

· Be careful once you have done this, as other things can rush to fill the void, for example other people's needs or demands or an old lover on the phone. Or you may feel uncomfortable and rush to fill up the space.

· Keep emptying the vessel, wait, hold still and when the true desire is ready, it will begin to unfold in a grounded, natural way.

Exploration: the Creative Process

To become more aware of this process in your life and when you are working on a creative project.

· Notice these stages in your creative life.

· Conception. Conceive an idea – do not tell others. Hold it and let it grow or make a conscious decision not to let it grow and let it go.

· Gestation. Anything is possible; you are nurturing, dreaming, resting and collecting your materials. You can often travel deeply into your own psyche. Be aware of the different levels and check out if you are getting swamped with old stuff instead of nourishing the creative idea.

· Labour. Challenging because now you need to work at it. If you begin this prematurely you may damage the creative seeds or cut off some promising new inspiration. But when you are ready. Toil. Sit down at computer and write day after day. Or paint. Or sculpt. Dance. Practise your healing art. Hone your craft. Learn how to do it. There are ups and downs. Here is where you need to remember the joy of the conception because the reality of the work may not seem to match your dreams.

· You may try to push it and try to birth before you have the groundwork done. Practise, practise.

· Energy can go down. You can feel defeated, depressed,

bored, repulsed and want to give up. Don't give up. A lot of people at this stage do not have the staying power, but you can get help and encouragement. When you meet the block you can have the support of others to help you through.

· Birth. You may not feel ready but your body is doing it. The baby is coming and there may be something wrong with it. You hope that you have completed all the previous stages adequately because now the baby is here and people are going to see it.

· This can be a confusing time. You are coming to an ending and old hurts and traumas can resurface; you may feel grief, rage, you may want to hide, nest or run away. Or it could all go smoothly – a nice, gentle homebirth with the time to enjoy it. Stay as centred in the stillness as you can. Dance to some safe, gentle music; nurture yourself.

· Rearing. Once you have the baby, you now have to rear it. Get it to the publisher/the art gallery, audition, decorate your healing room, advertise for clients. Put more energy in. Promote your project and see that it is recognised and yet guard that child against others' vague criticism or hostility.

· Now you must let that child go into the world. Here is where you are tempted once again to try and pull back and hold on but you must let this young creative adult go to other people who will relate to, be mean to, cherish, live with and create with it. As this happens, the creative dream opens out and becomes bigger than you. A play becomes different when it is interpreted by the actors. A book becomes something else in the mind of the reader. A painting may be loved or ignored by the people who come to view it.

· It is a sad time as you say goodbye, let go, and yet still keep in contact with it and there are many little deaths as old ways die to make room for the new. And at the same time another creative child is conceived and the whole process begins again.

· Be careful, do not try to have too many children; you may

not have the energy to rear them all. Be selective and only go with your deepest desires, your life path.

· Contemplate the words: conception – gestation – labour – birth.

· You can paint this if you like or use images to show these stages. You can take your time, spend weeks at it if you would enjoy this. Then put it in your bedroom and look at it every day without analysing or judging it. Just look at the images or colours you have made.

· When you are ready, move or dance conception, then gestation, labour and birth. Notice how these stages of the creative life process appear in your life.

· Note the stage you may be stuck in or the stages you thrive in. Use your images as a map that illuminates this and even though it will feel difficult, stay with the stages where you are weak and spend time nurturing these.

Exploration: Dance your Desire

· Move your tongue and taste the fluids in your mouth. Have you lost your taste for life? Does it feel dull, heavy, boring?

· Does it seem strange to move your hips? Is it sensual? Can you explore the sensations in your body?

· Do you feel a need to project your sensual energy or can you enjoy it yourself?

· Feel the base of your spine. Lean into each hip, loosen out. Close your eyes; feel into it.

· Now move your hips in a bigger way, drawing circles with the base of your spine.

· Breathe in and expand your belly. Pull the internal muscles upwards and inwards as you breathe out.

· Let the energy rise through your body.

One of our male dancers said this is not an easy movement for him because of his dangly bits! But men need to dance in the waters of their body, to receive sensual pleasure and to give it and to be given permission to sink down into this place without fear, guilt or the need to control.

· Make a treasure map of your desires or simply write them down. Now let your body move so you can dance that desire in your body. Let your body move, have paints ready and let that paint flow, don't censor, just let your body do it.

If we breathe in this orange light and work with the power of the creative process, miracles can happen. When we block it we feel the resistance and the pain. The key to unblocking is to create a safe, supportive atmosphere and have a willingness to contain the turgid emotions and use them to inform the dance or a song or poem. This allows that fizzy joy to bubble up...

Exploration: Gathering Energy
To gather dissipated energy and practise sensual movement and touch.

· Centre, pull back all of your energy from where you may be dissipating it or where you have allowed it to be stolen or given away by projecting it onto other people, worrying about them, or about bills, or spilling it out by talking too much about your creative energy and inner life.
· Sense into your hands. Let your hands be drawn to some-where on your body that needs massage or touch. Gently begin to massage your body. If you have aromatic lotions, then use these. Notice when you split off and begin to think and what part of your body you were touching when this happened. Work for just a couple of minutes at first and build on that every day.
· Now let your massage become a dance; an intimate dance with your own body. Close your eyes and let your hands see your body.

· If you start thinking, then stop and let the touch be gentle, simple. Go slowly, at your own pace. You may only be able to massage your hands and feet at first. Massage your wrists and your ankles; really get to know them.

Exploration: Water People
Seeing through sensual eyes.

· What would your water-man be like? Your water-woman? The women in the film *Monsoon Wedding* were water women for Jennifer; she loved their fluid eyes and lush bodies. The book *Chocolat* did it for Mark. Joanne loves the book *The Red Tent*; it inspires her as a woman. James thought the women in the film *Like Water for Chocolate* showed aspects of his inner female. Explore this for yourself; you are looking for sensuality and an ability to wait and meander and let things be. Not tuning into thoughts so much as tuning into atmosphere, sensation and sensuality. My water-man is able to take his time, sensually making love with a tender touch, able to use all his senses; he is aware of the flowing that goes on below words.
· Take time to commune with water. Connect with water – life, plants, fish, dolphins, seals and otters. Let their movements become your dance.

Let your eyes become soft and fluid and receive what you see. Instead of projecting your view outwards, gaze inwards.

Exploration: Mindfulness when Grooming
· Bring contemplation into your everyday grooming habits.
· Notice where you may avoid them or hurry through, with the thoughts driving you on.
· Pause; come into the moment, stay with the simple action

of brushing your hair, shaving, painting your nails or looking at yourself in the mirror.
· Put in the pause before the thoughts automatically comment.

Exploration: the Bowl of Sweetness

· In this place of receiving, this bowl, relax the whole area,
  let go of the terrible holding on in the lower belly, let go
  in the belly, the buttocks and genitals, you do not have to
  hold your tummy in; let it relax.
· Let the pelvis open slowly like a flower. Let your hands be
  sensitive as you touch your hips. Breathe; don't force, you
  are simply exploring.
· Sway your hips from side to side.
· Dip into this bowl of golden nectar with your breath.
  Looking inward, see the juices flow through the sacral
  area, the reproductive system and the genitals.
· This is life juice – let it gush through your lymphatic system and right through your body and into your skin.
· See it like oil softening your joints, muscles, and anywhere
  that feels stiff, sore or dry.
· See this juice gushing upwards from the sacral area
  through the body and cascading back downwards around
  the body and into the earth like a coloured fountain.

Exploration: Veiling and Mystery
To experience a sense of privacy, and respect for the inner mystery.

· Dance to the music of Sheila Chandra or original Egyptian
  music. Put on robes, veils and dark kohled eyes.
· Let go of any negative associations you may have with
  veiling and simply explore what it is to dance with veils or
  to wear long flowing garments.
· Dance to your own mystery. In our culture, it's all out
  there. Breasts and hips often thrust out aggressively. This

is a bowl and it is about receiving. It is also about containing – privacy and suitably veiling your inner mystery.
- Let your veil be blown by the breeze, tie ribbons to your ankles and wrists. Discover the privacy of shawls and robes and the experience of being wrapped in colour.

Exploration: Intimate Dance

Body awareness of the inner and outer, subtle boundaries and containment.

- Explore open movements and closed movements. Lie down and curl up foetus-like and then extend your limbs outwards like a starfish.
- Expand and contract your body.
- Explore advancing and then retreating by moving forwards and backwards. You can crawl, walk, slither.
- Strain forward to reach outwards and then pull backwards.
- Explore this with different body parts.
- See if you can find a midway place between reaching out and pulling inwards; between advancing and retreating; between open and closed movements. Put in the pause, breathe.
- If you are overactive in the sacral centre and inclined to act out your sexuality or emotions, or if you are looking for acceptance and love by giving to others, then use slow, inward movements and breathe gently.
- If you hold everything in your own inner space, then practise expanding the boundaries a little. Play with your hip movements and see what it is like to look outwards when you are dancing. Do all of this with breath and awareness.

Exploration: Dancing the Priestess/Prostitute

To rediscover the sacred female movements

- Dance like a prostitute. Move around the room as if you

were flaunting your body, move your hips, open your legs, really go for it.

· Now switch to being a high priestess making a big entrance in the sacred temple. Notice your movements. Notice where the split in your body is.

· Play with these movements; bring them together. Notice how they relate and what feelings come up when you bring together these two archetypes, both in their way equally frowned on by society and marginalised, they are also deeply connected in the body in a way you may discover for yourself.

· Dance these two now; move your hips, open your legs and see the swirling and snaking of the hips as sacred movements.

Exploration: Containers and Boundaries

· Use beautiful colours and smells, play soft music. This dance is about sensing into the most intuitive part of you – your deep belly. When you do this you know when to reach out, when to contain, when to be still and when to play. You learn how to rest deeply in the bowl of your own being and let everything flow from there.

· You give yourself permission to dance and to rest into the dance.

· When you are dancing, be aware of where your energy is contained in your belly and then explore this energy moving outwards towards someone else or some object in the room.

· What is the sensation like when the energy moves outwards. What happens in your third eye?

· Draw the energy back and feel the separation between you and the object or person. Breathe.

· As you go about your life, notice when your attention is caught up in other people, how they are behaving, what they are saying, or where you are being drawn into their energy field. Notice what happens. Have you lost a connection with yourself? Do you know how you are feeling, what you are thinking?

- Practise drawing your energy inwards by pausing and checking out your breath. You can gently undulate your hips in a small way so you can become centred again.
- Physical boundaries create psychic boundaries. If you become enmeshed emotionally, you become enmeshed in a pshchic way. Practise disengaging and communicating from a grounded, centred place. This creates intimacy.
- Buy a colouring book and some colours – any colouring book you are drawn to. In this way you learn about containers and boundaries.
- You can also buy a tracing book and trace images.
- You can colour in mandalas which are circle drawings/paintings that contain sacred images or sacred geometrical shapes or the energetic shape of a particular chakra; or you can create a mandala by drawing a circle on a page using a plate as a guide and then colour in your mandala using whatever shapes or colours you are drawn to spontaneously.
- If, on the other hand, you are self-absorbed and too completative, you may need to practise playing with and relating to others spontaneously. Or, if you are very structured, controlled and neat and unable to make a mess, use colour to make a mess on the page and allow the creativity to flow more. Play music and find a creative outlet – cooking or painting – that helps you to create without too much planning. Make up your own recipes, make a mess, try a little creative chaos.

Exploration: Rest is an Absence of Stimulation

The old fashioned GP would often recommend that a sick person should 'take a rest cure'. This rest would involve an absence of stimulation. Now we rest while watching TV or don't rest at all; just take the medicine and hope it will go away. This exploration is truly health-giving on every level.

· For one day, rest without stimulation – no phones, no radio, computer, TV, etc. No friends calling, no planning, no creating. Simply being.

· For health reasons I recommend that once a month you potter around your house, lie about, let your body move like a cat's and find the sunny spots or watch the rain. Simply sit and stare. Or dance to the rhythm of your own silence.

Exploration: Surrender

To help you to let go of the momentum and control that is often suppressing the female, creative energy.

· Close your eyes, notice where you are holding your body unnecessarily, let go of your breath, let go of everything.

· Notice if there is pressure pushing you forward or upwards

· Sink in to the sea of your body. Notice sensations in your belly and in the waters of your body.

· Let go and surrender to your body. Let your hips move slightly, and let your tongue move in your mouth.

· Let go of your thoughts and any momentum in the body.

· Surrender to the sounds around you. In this moment let it be safe for you to sense into your belly, let your wrists move and your ankles.

· Call on the female essence, pull back any wanting or trying; wait, listen, taste and touch.

· Open your mouth and let the sound come from your deep belly.

Exploration: Water Ritual

· Realise how powerful water is in your life. Notice the change in your body after a shower or a bath, even after washing your hands.

· Water has always been used for healing and ritual. Before a ritual, wash each other's feet, or go to the river as an act of faith and wash away your pain or a behaviour that is no longer serving you.

· Take time to acknowledge the sacredness of water; the holy wells and ancient rain.
· Sense the waters within you. Bless water before you drink. Bring water to your altar or before you dance and dedicate your dance to the healing of water on the earth and in your own body.
· When you are finished, drink that water mindfully.
· Put water in the sunlight. You can add to this by putting coloured gels around the glass of water so that the sunlight comes through that colour and into the glass. Store your coloured water in the fridge and sip a little in the morning and evening.
· Dance in the rain.

Exploration: Blindfold Tasting

You my know this game. Play it with children or on your own.

· Get some things to touch and taste: salt, sugar, honey, bread, chocolate, jelly, mushrooms, grated apple.
· Guide each other to the food, put your fingers on it, smell it, taste it. Take time to savour the touch and taste and see can you recognise it and experience it as new.
· Close your eyes when you are tasting food, water, air.
· Practise smelling and tasting. The scent of water and the female essence is subtle.
· Eat using your fingers instead of cutlery. The tips of the fingers are connected to our sense of taste and food from the fingers is more easily digested as we are using all our senses. The sense of touch, smell, sight, taste and even sound. What a feast!

Exploration: Orange Nectar

· See your pelvis as a bowl of orange liquid.
· You are slowly swirling this nectar in the bowl and containing it without spilling a drop.
· Make little sucking noises with your mouth and tongue.
· Wear soft, flowing garments. Don't fix your eyes on any one
thing, let your eyes be diffuse by gently taking in the whole
picture until the lines blur as your gaze turns more inward.
· Slowly move your hips. Draw all your juice back to your
pelvis and let it froth upwards through your body.
· Are you full of this life-giving energy or have you been
wasting it or letting it splash on dry ground, or on other
people who are not open to your creativity or sensuality?
· Pull it all back. Notice where it went.
· Enjoy the sensation of moving your hips and lower spine.
· Put your hands on your belly and lower spine. Move into
any stiffness that may be there.
· Make round movements. Curl up, open out, move in wavy
ways.
· Let your hips undulate, but stay grounded. Don't drift off
into thoughts. Let your hip movements become bigger,
wilder. Stay grounded in your tail. Walk with your legs
open and your hips swaying.

Exploration: Mother's Back Meditation

· Feel in your body what it would be like to be a small child
tied onto your mother's back.
· Your mother is a native woman who lives mostly in nature.
You can smell the herbs she uses for cooking, healing and
washing coming from her skin.
· You are wrapped up tight on her back and her gentle movements rock you as she walks. You can smell the campfire
and hear the background noises of people cooking, working
and talking. The sounds of birds and the resonance of your
mother's soft song come through her body into you. You

are secure. You are making gentle sucking noises with your mouth on your finger. Use images that are comforting to your body and that help you to feel cherished.

Exploration: 'Slow Down, You Walk Too Fast'

- Pretend you are on holidays while going about your every-day life.
- Pretend you are sight seeing and exploring when you walk or drive, looking out for interesting places to visit and different routes.
- If the sun shines through your window, sunbathe for five minutes
- Close your eyes and pretend that the water coming from your shower is coloured.
- Act like you are with a lover who admires everything about you.
- When you cook, prepare the meal as if someone you greatly admire was coming for lunch.
- Keep a notebook and some colours or a small watercolour set or colour markers. Keep it to hand and play with it when you are waiting for somebody or at a tea break.
- Write words in your notebook – anything at all – put in images or reduced photographs of your altar.
- Notice water people and earth people.
- Collect colours; cut out reds, then oranges, and stick them on different strips. You can cut up old paintings and combine the colours.
- Notice people moving, the meandering water movements, the water shapes people make and the spaces in between them.
- Take time to listen to the river, lake, stream, ocean or even that dripping tap.

Meandering

> The fruits, the colours, mesmerize me in a quiet rapture that spins through my head. I am entranced by colour. I lift an orange into the flat filthy palm of my hand and feel and smell and lick it. The colour orange, the colour, the colour, my God the colour orange. Before me is a feast of colour. I feel myself begin to dance, slowly, I am intoxicated by colour.
>
> Brian Keenan, *An Evil Cradling*

Leave space to do nothing. Go to places you have always wanted to go. These dreamtimes give you a chance to connect with the mystic within. If you listen to this part of you, it is like being in love because you are making love with your inner nature. You develop a language with the artist within so that you can communicate with yourself in ways that only you can really understand. Others looking at your art, your dance or your writing can be reminded of their own creative language and that is a great communication. Remember to have a sensual, intimate relationship with the core of your being as you meander through your days; your life will become sweeter and you will become grateful for the taste of each new day. Become the lover and the loved as the relationship between inner female and inner male becomes deeply intimate and balanced. He can learn to give her the nurturing time and the love that she needs and she can infuse him with her intuition, sensuality and love.

Exploring Yellow – Fire Dance: Chakra 3

Key words or clues: solar plexus, shins, forearms, digestion, assimilation/elimination; movements are straight and moving outwards.

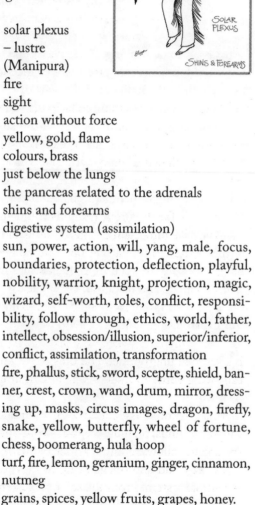

Third chakra	solar plexus – lustre (Manipura)
Element	fire
Sense	sight
Affirmation	action without force
Colours	yellow, gold, flame colours, brass
Location	just below the lungs
Endocrine gland	the pancreas related to the adrenals
Secondary chakras	shins and forearms
System	digestive system (assimilation)
Clues	sun, power, action, will, yang, male, focus, boundaries, protection, deflection, playful, nobility, warrior, knight, projection, magic, wizard, self-worth, roles, conflict, responsibility, follow through, ethics, world, father, intellect, obsession/illusion, superior/inferior, conflict, assimilation, transformation
Symbols and props	fire, phallus, stick, sword, sceptre, shield, banner, crest, crown, wand, drum, mirror, dressing up, masks, circus images, dragon, firefly, snake, yellow, butterfly, wheel of fortune, chess, boomerang, hula hoop
Fragrance	turf, fire, lemon, geranium, ginger, cinnamon, nutmeg
Food	grains, spices, yellow fruits, grapes, honey.
Discipline	healthy boundaries and self-worth, noble action,

	heroism, looking at fears of the mind, dissolving projections, judgements, attachments.
Issues	poor boundaries, shame, fearful thoughts, addictive/obsessive thinking, learning blocks, difficulty resolving conflict and being direct, busyness/workaholism, digestive problems, ulcers, hypoglycaemia, liver, pancreas, etc., depression, problems with adrenals/kidneys, overuse of force in one's actions and words, competitive, attacking, defending, inability to question one's own belief system.

When a man is awake, he exchanges energy with the hills and gives birth to a woman, an interior woman. When a man is asleep, his energy remains circulating inside himself and he gives birth to a machine.

Robert Bly

We prepare for the fire and sun dance by invoking the element fire. We tune into the solar plexus and feel the fire in there. Is it a small candle, a warm fire, a bonfire or a volcano? Does it feel relaxed as if the sun were melting it soft? Is there a glow of self-worth and a sense of grounded inner power, the lustrous gem, or Manipura, which is the Sanskrit word for this chakra? Is there a collapsing in the middle of the body as fear, shame, guilt and low self-worth eat away at the lustrous light? Or perhaps there is a sense of ungrounded grandiosity – 'I know it all'? Often we can swing between these two before finding a true sense of our own worth.

This chakra is associated with the male/active energy, the yang or animus, phallus, sceptre, sword and wand, the sun and the colour yellow. Yellow is associated with the intellect. It activates the mind and opens us up to new ideas. It also cleanses the whole system. From the solar plexus, the energy spins outwards; a deflector with the ability to deflect unwanted energy as we gain the power of discernment. It is also associated with the fire of digestion and assimilation which connects with our ability to digest our food and also our knowledge or information. The associated sense is sight, the way we see things, our perceptions and projections and the discernment to see through those.

When explaining this chakra we are assessing our ability to take action – to focus and to be disciplined; to mind our own business and to have appropriate boundaries with other people; to take in what we need and to deflect what is superfluous.

We are looking at our personal power and how that manifests in our body and energy body. The secondary chakras are in the forearms and shins. Other clues we have here are action without unnecessary force, autonomy, self-worth, roles and projection. We realise that we are mirrors and that we reflect at other people just as they reflect back at us and we track that energetically in the body through the different movements.

In this chakra, we also look at the fire of our digestive system, our ability to take in and assimilate, digest and let go. When we are healing this area, it is even more important to eat good food and not to overload the system.

If we have danced earth dance and fluid dance we can now draw from our rootedness and all that we have hatched in the dreamy belly and bring it forth through appropriate action. We meet the different roles and characters within our psyche and in the dance we explore roles, masks, magic and illusion. In this sun dance we are accessing our male energy. This is the energy you need to play chess, or to sword fight, some people love this energy, others recoil. At its best it is in the joy of playing together, the cut and thrust of it, the clash of swords as our sharpened will meets another's. Here is where you throw down the gauntlet, here is where you lay down the challenge. Here is where your sun power can finally begin to shine. It can be fun, the sound of the ball as it thwacks against the bat on a sunny day, the warrior initiation, or, it can be like the Fires of hell as the inner or outer conflict sets your thoughts alight and stings and burns you up. The quiet power of the male who has experienced life and his own inner nature, a person who knows all the games that people play, has given up judging and is radiating with warm, warrior, fire energy. Other people are drawn to this gentle but strong, male energy in the woman or the man, as they would be to sunlight or a glowing fire.

"Are you coming out to play?" This is the question we often ask ourselves in fire dance.

Music
Look for music that inspires the body to move the shins and forearms and affects the solar plexus and the warrior within. Here are some examples of music we have played with.

· Hero music, e.g. the theme from the films *Gladiator*, *The Last of the Mohicans*, *The Mission* or *Braveheart*
  Rousing music that stirs you out of lethargy. *Spartacus*.
  Or Native warrior music, e.g. *Sacred Spirit-Chants and Dances of the Native Americans* (New World Music, recorded anthology of American Music Inc.)
· Circus music. Marching music. The music of the cancan. Music for Jiving
· Music from the musicals, e.g. 'Yankee Doodle Dandee'.
· Songs like, 'The Lambeth Walk', 'My Old Man Says Follow the Band'
· National anthems to experience the quality of the music and where it resonates in the body
· Joseph Locke, 'We'll Make a Bonfire of our Troubles', Frank Sinatra 'My Way', Shirley Bassey, 'I am what I am'
· Ritual fire dance, Falla. *Radetzky March*, Strauss
· Vintage traditional jazz
· Rave music
· Father music: some of the tracks from Ayub Ogada or Baba Mal. (tender grounded male voices are very soothing, especially male voices singing in harmony or singing lullabies.)
· Children's songs, playful rhymes, stories and songs: 'The

Teddy Bear's Picnic', 'The Sun Has Got its Hat On', 'King Caractacus', Irish rhymes etc. Songs from children's musicals, e.g. 'I Just Can't Wait to be King', 'Mickey Mouse March'. 'Colonel Hathi's March' (The Elephant Song) – available from *Ultimate Disney CD*.

· And so much more. Research some for yourself!

The Colours Around You – Yellow

Yellow can be a good colour if you experience learning difficulties or blocks. The solar plexus is often called the brain of the nervous system; it feeds information to the brain and gives us gut messages about experiences we are having. It also extends out and checks out the environment around us. Too much yellow can make us feel spacey or forget our limitations. Lots of bright ideas, but perhaps they are unrealistic or not grounded. Used at the right time it can bring us clarity in our affairs so we can focus and be straight. Yellow is a good colour for cleansing, particularly for the liver and the intestines. Yellow activates the nervous system and the lymph glands. It helps with the elimination of calcium and lime deposits in arthritic conditions and is good for skin ailments. Gold especially activates the higher mental processes. It activates the motor nerves and therefore brings energy to the muscles.

Golden yellows give us a feeling of luxury. Use yellow with rose pink or blue to soften its effects. In her book, *The Power of Colour to Heal the Environment* Marie Louise Lacey says that the darker yellows and mustards can reflect badly on the complexion and that mustard yellow is associated with deviousness. Pale yellow can give a mental lift, but can also sap us of energy like a watery, winter sun.

Yellow is sun-like, active, energising and cleansing (use lemon in warm water first thing in the morning). Too much yellow overactivates the nervous system and we experience burn out. Sometimes it is the colour that stimulates us into action when we have been paralysed with worry. Remember how it affects the muscles.

In our houses it is a good colour for areas we are studying or active, but can be over stimulating if we need to rest or meditate. We have found that when we introduce yellow light, people become very chatty and witty but can overdo the talking and socialising or become overexcited and then feel drained later on, or they become very opinionated and argue a lot. So we balance the yellow light with soft rose pink and complementary blues. Violet and yellow together are very powerful; two cleansing colours. The violet ray of purification connecting with the higher will and the yellow of the gut and the will of the personality will, for most people be overwhelming, but it can be good if used by a colour therapist for certain diseases.

If you are afraid to extend yourself in the world, then yellow is a good colour to work with but not for people who are suffering from nervous exhaustion or in the early stages of recovery from an addiction. Instead use a rose pink or turquoise. If you are feeling low and lacking in self-worth, breathe an apple green colour into your solar plexus and breathe out any dingy colours. Surround yourself with yellow flowers or fruits, lemons and limes, pineapples, grapefruits, bananas, etc., or with copies of brightly coloured paintings like those of Gauguin and Van Gogh. Lemon oil is lovely to use around the house and can be combined with sea salt as a cleanser. Cleaning the bathroom, kitchen, fridge or worktops, it is a powerful disinfectant and leaves a lemony smell.

Put a yellow scarf around your solar plexus or wear yellow if it suits you. Or wear apple green, a combination of green and yellow, which is good for self-worth issues. Yellow can also be the colour of the coward or the addictive controller or the person who is obsessed with their own belief system, thoughts and illusions. In these cases, the yellows around the person are often dingy or there is a startling bright yellow and not enough of the softer, kinder colours.

Yellow is stimulating. It can act as a laxative and is a highly potent cleanser. Good to use in the spring or autumn for a detox. Do not meditate with this colour before bedtime or use it in your bedroom because it will keep activating your thoughts and you may find yourself waking and thinking immediately about work you have to do that day. Or you will be going over conversations and ideas you had during the day and hopping up in the middle of the night to use the loo because the overactivity will be affecting your kidneys. It is the perfect colour for morning and morning is the time for the yoga postures that make up the asana to the sun or a time to breathe in the sunlight through the solar plexus. This is very good for people who suffer from depression in winter, as is fire dancing. Sunflowers and sunflower seeds are full of sun, as are grapes and other fruits.

Yellow is for activity, mental alertness, new ideas, focus, clarity and self-worth. Check out your wardrobe and the colours in your home. If you are using a lot of yellow, you have a good mind but probably need more rest time, so perhaps add the colour pink for relaxation and tenderness for your self and all that you do. If you are sluggish and prone to being stuck or fearful and unable to motivate yourself, then add golden yellows onto the walls in your kitchen or hall and that will have an effect. If you are in the early stages of recovery from any kind of addiction or suffering with nervous exhaustion, then do not use yellow; use turquoise and soft pink and later on begin to introduce the colour in a small way, for example in a candle, a flower or a piece of soft cloth. Use soft, glowing yellows that have a touch of pink in them.

Exploration: Basic Movements

- Play with these movements now. Check your posture, open out your legs and soften your knees and find a good sense of balance. Check that your pelvis is not thrust forward. Sit down into your hips.
- Bring forearms away from the solar plexus, keeping your hands straight, and explore the space around you.
- When you have warmed up sufficiently, begin to move in straight lines and diagonals through the space you are in. Focus your eyes on a place in the room and move towards

it in a direct line leading from your solar plexus, forearms and shins.

· Experience the contrast between moving through the space in curving pathways and with round movements as we did in the last colour.

· You can try kicking and blocking with your forearms and shins as you move around the space.

· If you are inclined to force your energy outwards or inclined to rush at things or be over-competitive, the movements need to be T'ai Chi-like, hips low, knees soft.

· Let the joints be loose – no force. Throw out your arms like a rag doll. You are looking for action without force, movement without force, but there can be a little tension in the muscles.

· You can play around with this. If you are always holding back, afraid to put your energy out there or not able to maintain boundaries, move forward and make stabbing movements with a stick. Check that you are moving forward with your legs and not leaning over at the waist.

· Extend your energy outwards. Expel sharp sounds from the solar plexus, 'Ha! Hee!'

· Let your breath be easy and don't tighten up the body; it needs to be loose, flexible and accurate.

· You also need to be grounded and not out of balance in the base. True warriors need to be able to stand still, totally relaxed and alert with good peripheral vision, in tune with their breath and the rhythm rising up through them. Then they can move easily without losing energy by unnecessary forcefulness. If they lose presence, become distracted and pause to think or ponder on a matter, they will quickly lose ground and may be lost. You are looking for total presence here.

Exploration: Create an Altar

- To make your fire altar: mirrors are good, rulers, a boomerang, a camera, warrior pictures, symbols and images.
- One dancer had deer antlers on hers, another an old sword. You could use a banner with the name of your project, or coloured festive flags.
- Pictures and images associated with fiesta, play, carnivals, circuses, masks and street theatre are good.
- Sunflowers, daffodils and images that conjure up magic for you and the warrior or wizard energy.
- If you are feeling confused and overwhelmed, then the colours rose and gold and one single object can bring about a sense of stillness and focus.

Exploration: Roles

- What are the roles you play in your life? Dance these.
- How does it feel in your body? Is your body grounded? What sensations are in your tummy?
- What role would you like to play? Dance this and notice sensations in your body.
- Who are your role models, your real heroes? Who do you aspire to be like?
- Collect pictures and put them on your wall or in a scrapbook.
- Try on these bodies. What does it feel like to move like one of your heroes?

Exploration: Motivators

- Why do you do things? Look at your life, at the projects you are planning or the work you are doing. Ask the question: Why am I doing this? What motivates me? Do not give a quick answer; let the question rest there.
- Make a list and see what motivates your actions, e.g. I go swimming on Mondays because Mary does and I want

her to like me. Or, I am cleaning my house so people won't think badly of me. Or, I have a career as a doctor because I find out now that this was always my father's secret wish for himself. Or, I am doing this work because it will earn me some money and I can buy the food and clothes I need and like. Or, I am not doing my housework today because I need to paint and painting makes me sing inside.

· How do you make decisions? Are you decisive/indecisive? Should have done this? Should have done that? What do you need to make a decision about right now, what is motivating you to make this decision? Do you often set up decisions for yourself between two courses of action? How long do you spend mulling over these decisions and how much of your energy is used?

When our actions are driven by our fear, the fear increases, or, desires that come from unconscious conditioning keep pushing us forward, causing more fear and lack of rest. When we discover the hidden motives behind our actions, we often find that we do not have to do so much and our actions arise from a gentler source.

Exploration: Focus

· Put your focus on all the good in your life and on all your good qualities. Every day, take time to focus on these and on the progress you are making.
· If you have a problem, focus on all the good things you are learning as you deal with this. Dance this, drum this and sing it.
· Notice your posture when you acknowledge the good. Notice it when you are besieged with negative thoughts.
· Focus on the people who encourage you and who give you a warm feeling in your solar plexus.
· If you are inclined to be a people pleaser/co-dependent,

take time everyday to focus on your own business and what your priorities are. Notice when you are focusing on other people's business.

· If you are already inclined to do this and have a tendency to be introverted and not move towards others, focus on ways that you can send your energy outwards. Connect with others who are on a similar journey or who are working with their creativity; ring them up and make a date for coffee or lunch. Be prepared to deal with rejection, but don't take it personally; maybe they really are too busy. Look around for someone who might be willing to make the connection; local writers' or artists' groups, a café.

Remember – what you focus on *grows*.

Exploration: Building Energy

· Dance down in the base, move from one foot to another slowly, keeping the rhythm. Stay in one place, but focus on something at the other side of the room.

· Begin to build on the energy coming from the earth. When you feel the animal power moving through your body and you are staying in rhythm and are well balanced, begin to hop from one foot to the other one-two, one-two. Let the energy build right through your body, don't move too quickly. Wait until you have a nice steady rhythm that you could stay with for a long time – wait – wait – wait.

· Now, keeping the rhythm, begin to advance towards your goal – your focus at the other side of the room. At this stage, a lot of people lose the rhythm or they try to move too quickly and lose energy. If this happens, you will quickly lose your breath and the top of your body will be ahead of your feet. Your rhythm will have speeded up. Go back to the beginning and build slowly.

· When we do this in groups, we often divide the group into two and we become warriors advancing as if for battle, with the other group standing their ground and watching us advance. We make faces and sounds like warriors of old. It's great fun it is also very powerful.

· If you can work with your energy and power and advance across the room in a steady, balanced way, what does it feel like when you arrive? Notice these feelings in your body, not in your imagination.

· Be like a tiger, paced, fluid, and powerful. Feel your paws, your strong jaw and your haunches propelling you forward.

· Now explore the other side of that, the dipping of your foot in the water and retreating. The moving forwards, then cowering back. Play with it.

· Be the old battle-worn tiger, moving through your territory. You may have been through a lot and you may be tired and old, but you've got the eyes and the experience that younger cubs don't have. You don't have to waste too much energy. Your moves are subtle, practised. You know when to rest up and when to *move*.

Fear in the solar plexus

In the solar plexus, we feel a different kind of fear – fear of the mind.

Exploration: Map your Fear

· Get a large sheet of paper and some old magazines, scissors and Pritt stick.

· Select images and words at random that symbolise your fears around becoming more creative or beginning a new project.

· Really go for your worst fears and put them out there where you can look at them.

Exploration: Who Do You Feel Superior To?

· Notice who you feel superior to and who you feel inferior to.

· Notice where the sensation is in your body. Don't try to do anything with it or change your thinking, simply notice.

· You can also dance these sensations and you can dance as the people you feel superior to and the people you feel inferior to.

· Notice how that feels in the body.

· Look at the person you feel inferior to. Now ask yourself this question: has this person got more knowledge than I have or are they better at something I would like to be good at?

· If so, why not acknowledge them for their gifts and ask them to support you as you learn – be careful, are you trying to impress them or learn from them?

· Now look at the person you feel superior to and see if you are acknowledging their power. Look for power in them and acknowledge this.

· Why are you feeling superior? What measuring ruler are you using? More intelligent? Does intelligence measure the worth of a person? Better looking? Better breeding? More money? More evolved? More privileged? A harder worker?

· Write down or make a collage of your own belief system. Who taught you this? On what basis are you making your judgements?

Exploration: Hahhhh

- Watch all of your movements. Slow them down. 'I am raising my arm', or, 'I am breathing in a shallow way and my head is bending forward'.
- Notice the way the thoughts want to speed it up or how they can become impatient: 'This is boring'.
- Hold that and let your body move. With your eyes softly focused, let your forearms lead the movement. Your hands are straight, karate-like, fiery fingers, protecting your solar plexus, but also exploring the air all around this area, front and back.
- Your movements are direct, sharp and clean.
- Let your eyes be diffuse so you are taking in the whole room without focusing on one thing. In this way you have peripheral vision which makes you a better warrior.
- Bring in some kicks and make the sound 'Hah' from the solar plexus. If you are a quick, impatient person, let the sound be long and soft, 'Haaaaaaaaaaa'.
- Hold your sword or spear with two hands above the body. Notice your body in space. Where is your pelvis? Where are your shoulders? Are your legs soft and secure with a good, warrior stance?
- Try these movements in front of a mirror. Are you collapsing in the middle? Is your pelvis thrust out? Where are your shoulders?
- Do not try to change your body, but really sense into how this feels. Notice your knees. What effect is this way of standing having on the energy in your body?
- Ask your body to show you a way to come into alignment.

Exploration: Childhood Games

- Use a big sheet of paper and coloured markers. Divide the paper into sections age 0-5 yrs 5-10 yrs and so on. In each section describe and name the games you played.

· Notice at what age you stopped playing and why. What or who replaced this? In what ways do you play now?

NB In one group this particular exercise brought up a lot of pain for a man who never had the chance to play. If this is your experience then find a good person to work with, one to one.

Exploration: Throwing
To practise deflecting unwanted energy and other people's projections on you. Also to notice where you are sending out your energy and thoughts inappropriately.

· Stand easy on flexible legs, knees slightly bent. Use a cushion or pillow, throw from the solar plexus at the wall and let out a 'HAH' sound.
· Now go and collect the cushion and pull it in towards the solar plexus and make a comforting sound.
· Practise throwing it away and letting the energy go with the 'hah', pulling the energy back in with the cushion.
· Notice your arms and hands and the way you grip the cushion. Notice your legs, notice where you are holding back around the shoulders or upper arms, become as relaxed as you can.
· Don't worry about what this is for, just do it and notice any changes in your body or way of being.
· If you are inclined to quick anger, then practise dancing this but slow everything down. Hold the cushion for longer, notice what happens when you pick up the cushion and bring it in towards your solar plexus. Notice your legs when you are throwing it.
· Breathe and stay as conscious as you can.
· Be deliberate in your actions. Let your voice come.
· If you are yelling and hitting out, notice, listen, whose voice is that? Whose action? What other sensations are in your body? What is going on in your legs and feet?

· Have some paper and crayons ready. Now let your hands draw on the paper then dance what you have drawn.

Exploration: Energy Ropes (working in twos and working with boundaries)

· Play this with a friend. You are pulling an energy rope connecting to his solar plexus. Pull him slowly towards you. Your partner goes with this, experiencing all the sensations in the solar plexus until you are up close to each other.
· Now swap over and have your partner pull you in.
· Now put on sacral music and dance, containing the energy in your hips and solar plexus.
· Dance together, coming close together and moving apart.
· Practise containing your energy as you do this
· Now work with pulling on each other's energy ropes. You can practise by using ropes in sacral, solar and heart.
· Are these familiar sensations?
· Take time to paint these sensations and let words rise up

Exploration: Making the Shield and Working with Boundaries

· Making the shield does not have to be the greatest art in the world nor does your dance have to be a perfectly executed warrior dance in symbol and shape. Find the materials from whatever you can gather. You can drop the accumulation of defensive armour you built up over the years and be protected by a paper shield and a toy sword, a symbol of the light energy in the body.
· When you make your shield, take your time; use pictures from magazines, crêpe paper, gold and silver paper, small mirrors (deflectors). Your intention is to let go of your rigid, armoured body and create a subtle, flexible boundary.
· Trust your intuition. Go for pictures or words that may not even seem relevant. Use lots of colours and decorations.
· Put your shield somewhere you can see it every day.

Exploration: Fire Breath

- Breathe as if you were a dragon and your breath could be expelled from the solar plexus in a shooting flame.
- Pull in your solar plexus as you shoot out the flame and let a sound come.
- This can make you dizzy, only do what is comfortable.
- Hold your hands palms outwards in the region of your solar plexus. Push the energy outwards and move around, looking at your boundaries. Keep your knees soft, stay relaxed. WATCH YOUR BACK!
- Breathe slowly in through your mouth and out through your nose. Eyes soft.
- Then reverse: breathe slowly through your nose and out through your mouth. Soft eyes.
- Fill the air around you with your fiery breath.

Exploration: Hero Dance

- At some stage when you have integrated some of your shield work, play hero music, for example from the films *The Last of the Mohicans*, *Gladiator* or other Hero music that you can relate to.
- Or dance with no music and make fire sounds yourself. Hold your shield and your sword and DANCE.
- If you are feeling scared, use this music and call up the hero within. Move around the room, crouch low – get ready to spring. Clear the air around you – FIGHT!

Exploration: The Bellows

· Lie down, put some books on your solar plexus and breathe in, pushing your stomach out and raise the books.
· Now, slowly and gently exhale, lowering the books.
· Repeat for as long as is comfortable.
· Let your solar plexus be like a bellows blowing the fire. A weight on the solar plexus and consciously breathing and strengthening the muscles here definitely helps with fear and boundary work and the ability to project energy in a healthy way or protect one's own energy.

Exploration: Making Faces, Warrior Dancing

This exploration is for people who are afraid of conflict, not for those who habitually challenge and argue with others.

· To intimidate your enemy, practise pulling frightening faces, e.g. sticking out your tongue and rolling your eyes.
· This is great fun with a group of children. Think of tribal warrior dances.
· Dance around the fire. It might only be a business meeting, but if you are quaking with fear before that office bully you need to practise warrior dancing.
· Let the sounds come, sharp and strong: 'HA HEE HO'.
· How fierce can you be? Is your whole body fierce or are you wimping at the shoulders?
· Let your shoulders relate to your hips and pelvis. Let the tail swing like a cat's, remember the feminine energy and now the warrior defending his lady.
· What are you scared of? Become that. Make faces – hoo hoo, like a scary ghost. Play with the fear.
· Dance the predator then the prey. Let your face dance.
· Good music for this is fire drumming with a good slap to the drum that breaks up the stuck, stagnant, ghosty fear around the solar plexus. Or classical pieces Holst's *The Planets*, or the music of Rachmaninov.

Exploration: Sun and Moon Walks
Exploring and balancing the different energies yin/yang, solar/sacral, sun/moon.

- Walk as you would normally without trying to adjust yourself. Now walk as if you are on a beach, you are on an extended vacation and you have rented a little cottage, money is not an issue right now and you are free to meander on the shore. You watch the sun go down and the moon coming up. The waves lace around your feet. You are collecting seashells and dreaming of a creative idea you have had at the back of your mind for a long time.
- It could be a book, or a garden, a painting, a business idea, a song, music, basket-making, felt-making, restoring furniture, collage, whatever. You are gently dreaming this up, but also enjoying your evening stroll.
- Walk this, feel what it is like in your body. Use the picture fully and add into it. You might be strolling up to the local inn. Walk this, then dance it.
- Now picture this: You actually wrote your book, made your baskets, etc. and, in the process, you were deeply healed, you visited many dark places within, it was messy like any birth, but you did it. You put it out there and now a big publisher has expressed an interest or an art gallery or gardening programme, fancy shop – fill in the blanks. They want you to come to the city and discuss terms.
- You need to pack now. What will you wear? Book your ticket and so on. Notice the sensations in your body.
- You are in the city. You are dressed in your business clothes, you have been advised financially and you know that if you can get this deal it could mean you could live in that cottage and begin another creative project. There is a lot of traffic, people on mobile phones, you are on the street where the business contacts live, you are walking towards the building. You are psyching yourself up.
- Walk this, get to feel what it is like in your body, the

mounting excitement or dread, fear or power in the solar plexus. Notice the way you are walking. This is a part of yang male energy. Get to know it, make friends with it. Dance it.

· Change back to yin or moon, sacral energy back down on the beach in the moonlight, then change again, yang, sun energy, striding through the crowds. Notice the transitions. Notice are these two energies warring against each other or can they complement each other?

· These are two extremes, but even so they give a sense of what it is like to be inward-looking and reflective and to be out in the hustle and bustle interacting with other people.

Exploration: Dance your Sun and Moon Energies

· Let your body dialogue with these different ways of being.

· Notice the resistance as you move from one element to another, the water and then the fire.

· These two elements can put each other out or we can use the fire to heat the water, the water to cool the fire.

· See where you can sense these elements in your body not just in the belly or solar plexus, but how they dance right through the body burning through your heart or in your head – they can go out of balance or work in balance.

Exploration: Power

· Practise focusing on other people's power while still holding your own.

· When your thoughts automatically go to put someone up or down, hold the space, notice what happens physically in your body.

· Put in the pause before you put yourself down.

· Notice if you put someone up there – how later on you may have to pull them back down.

Marching

The movement of marching, all sorts of marching, stimulates the solar plexus and helps to discipline it. It is not so much chest out, quick march, as solar plexus out, quick march. If you have this knowledge you can use it for good. Practise marching and focusing the eyes straight ahead. Then eyes left – about turn, and march, then eyes right, about turn, and march. My mother used to use marching to help discipline the bodies of the children in her dance class so that they could coordinate their right and left-hand sides and learn to dance together. It also works to help coordination and right-left ability. The raising of the legs strengthens the muscles and the swinging of the arms moves energy through the body. Of course because of associations with armies, we may be wary of this way of moving because of its effect. Try it for yourself and see the effect on your body and mind. Put on Strauss' *Radetzky March* or other marching music and practise marching. Notice how you are moving. Put on circus music or dance with pom-poms, cheerleader style. In the solar plexus you find the energy to fly your flag. When we let go of associations with brass bands and armies, etc., we can come upon the simple pleasure of the child running after the big band as it marches down his street. Or the need to run away with the circus when they parade through the town. Put on 'Yankee Doodle Dandee' and tap-dance or do your version of a tap dance. That old top-hat-and-cane routine that Fred Astaire did so well. Other movements here are the charleston or the high kicks of the cancan. Get out that old jive music or the dances you used to do to showbands. Juggle with balls. Obviously you need to work up to these activities, but sense into them with your body and use that energy and dance a doodle of these kinds of movements so you get the idea.

Dance through the other elements and then see if you can sense the full connection between the three first chakras, rooting downwards, spinning inwards and then projecting outwards. This takes practise.

Exploration: a Treasure Map

- Make a treasure map. Tune in and ask for clarity. Trust what you choose in a random way.
- Now cut out pictures and words to create the life you would like to be living in a year's time.
- Put this treasure map on your wall and look at it every day.
- If there is one particular thing you need to manifest, like a house or a course, put up a picture of it and a picture of yourself as well and focus your energy on it every day.
- You can also put up your fear collage and hang your shield and sword beside it, also as one dancer did, you could veil it in tulle, in the pink colour of unconditional love.

Exploration: Fiery Man/Woman

- What sort of a man or woman do you know who could represent your warrior man or warrior woman?
- A fiery man or a fiery woman quick to act or with a temper.
- Do you know someone who can handle this solar plexus energy very well, a person who has good boundaries but a glow about them that people want to be near?

Exploration: Make a Magic Wand

- Gather sticks, feathers, shells, beads, string, berries, conkers, whatever you can find – to make your magic wand.
- You can use your pen as a magic wand. Tie a little feather on it so that you can see the powerful instrument it is.
- See your body as a magic wand. You can point your two fingers and change the air around you.
- Feel that power. Know that it is there and that you need guidance, support and a lot of practise in order to use it wisely.
- Never use your magic on another person. Leave every person to be autonomous and free. Use your magic to heal and create yourself. Then others will just want to come and

play, free to do so on their own terms. Then you can hold a space for them or assist them as they do their own healing. Now there are two magic wands and you can stand back and be amazed.

Exploration: Eye Games

· Close your eyes. Sense into your eyes and feel them soften and draw back into the sockets.
· Look inwards towards the back of the skull, upwards to the top of the skull and then into the third eye region (that space in the middle of the brow).
· Now look down towards your chin, then down and into your heart.
· Hesitate at each point for a second or for as long as feels comfortable.
· Now look into your solar plexus. Finally, look through the soles of your feet.
· Open your eyes slowly. Let your eyes roam around the room and notice what objects you focus on. Gently disengage. Let your eyes travel up towards the ceiling and down towards the floor. BREATHE. Now let your eyes travel over to the sides of the room and the corners.
· Focus outside the room letting your eyes travel over a tree or the sky – BREATHE – now gently come back and close your eyes and begin to focus within.
· All the time you are reminding yourself to breathe and keep your eyes softly focused.
· When walking outside, let your eyes trace the outline of a tree or a bush. Indoors look at the space in between objects and trace that space. Let your eyes move and allow your body to follow.
· If you are feeling fearful and obsessing about a particular person or situation this exercise can really help you to disengage.

If we refuse to let go of old ways of being, controlling and manipulating, then life will keep presenting these issues to us and we will experience strong sensation in the solar plexus as we prepare for change and the action required. There is also a lot of control here and fear, so it can feel overwhelming. Slow everything down. Accept your life as it is now. Dance that acceptance and also the fears; when the energy gets overwhelming it can freeze you and you won't feel like moving at all. Stay with those sensations and let your dance be tiny – you do not have to force the change, even though you may have been able to see it ahead of time. Let your body catch up, stay simple. Ask for help.

The solar plexus can get over-excited, terrified or we can pick up so much that it gets jammed and our nervous system gets overloaded. Take time to breathe soft colours into this area and empty out all the images, noises and roles. Use the affirmation 'no drama is good drama'. Slowly move your hands over the air around your solar plexus, smoothing, calming and clearing. Allow there to be emptiness. Like those wooden sculptures that have no middle. Let the breeze pass through. As we let go of the roles, opinions and thoughts, we empty our solar plexus and begin to tap into the vastness of the solar system that lies behind our projections. As we get more accomplished at this, we become less serious and know that a sense of play is absolutely necessary. Probably the best advice on how to heal the solar plexus would be – do what brings you fun, do what you enjoy most, do it alone and do it with those you love.

EXPLORING GREEN – HEART DANCE: CHAKRA 4

Key words or clues: Heart, chest, lungs, elbows, knees, respiratory system, circulatory system. Movements inwards and then extending outwards.

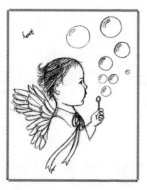

Fourth chakra	heart – unbound
Element	air
Sense	touch
Affirmation	'I tune into the rhythms of my heart. I open to life, I am simple and free.'
Colours	green, pink, rose, gold.
Location	centre of the chest, cardiac plexus, related to upper back, shoulders, breasts, arms, hands, lungs
Endocrine gland	thymus
Secondary chakras	elbows, knees, palms of hands, soles of feet
System	respiratory system – circulatory system.
Clues	touch, tenderness, mystery, veiling, privacy, beloved, compassion, hugs, space, humility, breath, receiving, inner child, balance, rhythm, flexibility, rigidity, frozen, simplicity, grief, sorrow/joy hearth, home, yearning, intimacy, romance, integration/ male/female, marriage, freedom/attachment, friendship, surrender, gratefulness, courage, miracles
Symbols and props	key, circle, feather, bird, wings, heart shapes, mobile, lace, gold, trinkets, roses, star, bell, cloud. mist, fog, veils, ribbons, balloons, bubbles, kite, wishing well, wishing chair.
Fragrance	rose, geranium
Food	herbs, cabbage, leafy green vegetables, green foods

Discipline	letting go, balance, able to receive and give
Issues	inability to receive and give love or feel compassion, unacknowledged grief, jealousy, resentment, disappointment, disconnection, rigidity, frozen, separation, heart disease, breast pain, lumps, cysts, have a heart, open heart, disheartened, coldhearted, heart of gold, heavy heart, light heart, divided heart

When my love comes and sits by my side, when my body trembles and my eyelids droop, the night darkens, the wind blows out the lamp, and the clouds draw veils over the stars.

It is the jewel at my own breast that shines and gives light.
I do not know how to hide it.

Rabindranath Tagore

We prepare to enter the heart by attuning with the element air. We begin in silence as we meditate on the heart chakra. The air often seems to turn misty like soft rain or fog as old grief rises to be cleared. Our attention may be drawn to the upper back, the shoulders, the thymus, chest, breasts, and our throat and jaw. We notice the joints particularly our knees and elbows. We may notice how rigid we feel in our upper back or chest - the lack of flexibility -There may be pain there - There may be a frozen, numbed out or shivery sensation in the heart area, front or back or simply a strong sensation.

Before we can enter the heart, really enter it, not a false sentimentality but to become truly intimate, we need to establish our boundaries first. It needs to be safe. Good work in Fire dance addressing issues in our relationships allows for deeper entry into our hearts and the openness to receive and become truly intimate. It is possible to love the other without invading them, allowing appropriate space and privacy in our relationships. Here in this green place where the colours yellow and blue combine to give us green, we are looking for the balance between the warm, earthy colours and the cooler blues. We focus on breath, lungs, rhythm, heart and the pulse of blood moving through our veins as we become aware of our circulation on every level: our need for privacy and rest and the need to circulate and be in relationships with others. We might wish to be light – to open our arms, to soar and fly, to laugh and play – and yet below this, another layer feels rigid, tired and heavy. We may be acting as if we are having a good time but underneath this high energy, the heart is low. The deeper we go, the more we come to the denseness that is occluding the light at the centre. By accepting this and allowing our bodies to be the way they are, it can feel safer and easier to come fully into this heart energy and the element air.

Music

Uillean pipes, tin whistle, low whistle, natural flutes and whistles, pan pipes of Peru, Native American flute, bird flutes, wind instruments etc.

Irish slow airs artists: Davey Spillane- *The Sea of Dreams* – Sony pure heart music, good for easing grief. Also oisinmcnally@ yahoo.com

- Tim Wheater, *Heartland* – toning choral piece. Cathartic-transformative, powerful
- Henryk Gorecki's *Symphony No. 3*, *Symphony of Sorrowful Songs*, transcending deep, unbearable grief also good in the crown chakra.
- Mahler's, *Love and Grief*
- Strauss, *The Blue Danube* and other waltzes – moving into lighthearted joy.
- Tchaikovsky, *Swan Lake*, *The Sleeping Beauty*
- Mozart, *Theme from Elvira Madigan*
- Chopin's *Nocturnes*
- John Field's *Nocturnes and Sonatas*
- Theme music from the film *The Piano*, Michael Nyman

Virgin Records (wonderful for dance and exploring
levels: high-low-middle-advance-retreat and different
atmospheres)
· 'Gabriel's Oboe' from *The Mission* Ennio Morricone, Virgin
Records, for heart dance – centering, coming home
· *Gospel Greats* – Various. Music that invites you to clap and
sing along, exploring gratefulness and exuberance.
· There are many more heart songs and melodies that you
can explore for yourself. Pick the ones that speak to you.

The Colours Around You – Green

The green ray affects the heart and the thymus gland. Green
soothes and relaxes and being in the green of nature helps us
to feel the space within our hearts. The green in nature helps us
to breathe and let go of build-ups in the system (overexposure
to radiation, e.g. mobile phones, computers, photocopiers, geo-
pathic stress) and overwhelm the energy field.

If we are grieving, nature within and around us can speak very
deeply to us – but people who are very shocked and unable as
yet to come towards their hearts will not like green and will shy
away from the colour or may become angry if you try to bring
them towards it. The green ray is the harmoniser, the balance
between heaven and earth. It brings peace, balance and harmony.
The different shades are associated with different states. Bright
clear summer greens indicate a clear, loving heart, enthusiastism
and openness to life. Dark greens indicate strength and maturity.
Sometimes the dark green can be a strong, earthy colour. When
I came out of a long relationship I adored a green wool jumper
that had been dyed with a natural earthy dark green. It was like
lying by a river that was overhung with weeping willows and
dark evergreens with sunlight dappling through. Its wet soggy
colour was like lying in moss. I could even imagine these soggy
greens being applied like wet herbs to my hurt heart. Olive
greens and sage greens help us to relax and digest, as do the
greens of autumn fruits. Dark, stagnant greens can show us old,

stuck, glucky emotions that need to be cleansed and cleared, or old deceit and jealousy lying brooding there and old hurts and wounds that may be festering. Green affects the digestive system (the ability to take in and let go). It is an excellent colour for shock, particularly when used with its complementary colour, magenta. In colour therapy, green has no true complementary colour, but it works very well with magenta. It helps to polarise and balance the whole system. Breathe green in horizontally into the chest area and magenta in through the soles of the feet and the crown of the head. Green is an excellent tonic for the lungs. Eat green leafy vegetables, avocadoes, grapes, etc. But particularly the leafy vegetables for the heart and lungs or drink juices made from spinach, cabbage and sage. Green regulates blood pressure – light green for high blood pressure, dark green for low blood pressure. My teacher, Marie Louise Lacey, used to say that if someone had cancer, green was often missing from the aura. I have had experience of this personally by finding a subtle resistance to the colour when healing a breast lump and with clients who were working with malignant tumours in this area. Often green can bring up too much grief for the person to bear. If the heart is in acute pain, then use rose pink and the symbol of the mystic rose. Green is also the colour we need to heal any circulation problems we might have, a resistance or fear of moving and circulating with others, or a resistance to being part of the community. Paradoxically, too much involvement in the community and not enough nurturing of self can lead to cancer and heart attacks or heart-related illnesses, e.g. high or low blood pressure, strokes, losing the heart for life, disheartened, exhausted. If you find it hard to wear green, then wear turquoise or put green leafy plants around your house or soft green velvets and when you are walking, feel the green colour coming into you from the air and the trees. Ask the colour green to support and help you heal your heart and also the soft rose-gold to let go of past hurts.

Exploration: Connecting with your Heart

· Dance through the other energy centres to become as fully grounded as you can.

· When the intention alone or in a group is to come into relationship with your heart, your awareness will move there, but make sure you dance right through the physical body first and stay in the base; otherwise you may become too airy and space out.

· Let the heels beat out a rhythm on the earth and let a sound come in your chest – 'hahahahah' – punctuate it with your heels gently bouncing on the ground.

· Notice breath. Move shoulders and upper body, search into rigid or stiff places.

· Take time to release jaw, neck and face.

· Stay with your breath. Push into arms and upper arms, push into the heels of your hands – flex your elbows and roll your shoulders.

· Keep tracking sensation in your body. If you are hunched over, dance this hunched-over dance.

· Slow it down, stay with it for as long as your breath allows.

· If your body is stiff or cold, then dance this stiffness or coldness, go with it, become it and let it express itself through the dance. Let your body shake. Let the little groans, moans or bigger sounds come through you. Listen…

· You may wish to choose some music, the Irish slow airs seem to speak to a heart place within us – you can find music that soothes this area of your body.

· Listen to music and see where in your body the music or song resonates. Sometimes you intuit just the right music and it can serve as the key. Or you might read an old fairy story or have a dream and you could dance to that dream.

· Hold upper arms until they ease out and release, touch upper arms, back and chest tenderly.

· Be careful not to lose your connection to the base, hands and feet or the movements can become ungrounded.

· Notice if you are being sentimental instead of authentic in your movements.

Exploration: Rose – Heart

In this dance you are allowing habitual movements and defences to dissolve while rediscovering the potential for gentle heart movement and sensitive touch. We play Davey Spillane's 'Equinox', a slow instrumental, for this.

· Kneel, sit or lie. Begin with no movement, simply becoming aware of your breath, heartbeat and the blood moving through your body.
· Let little fingers move and then one by one let other fingers join in, then the hands, wrists and lower arms.
· Notice your capacity for movement, how even the little fingers can dance.
· You can have music playing or move to silence and your own heartbeat.
· Allow the air to move your hands and arms. If your arms get tired, you are putting in too much force. Rest and begin again.
· Sustain the movements as if you are pushing the air, then let arms float.
· Try cradling movements or reaching outwards and then coming back and holding your heart. Move arms to the back and side.
· Keep the movements slow, but stay grounded. You are noticing sensations, but keep movements physical. If you see colour or images, allow them to be there but come back to the physical movement.
· Explore the air. Notice how far you can reach into all the space around you. Change the quality of your movement – sometimes light airy, sometimes firm – as you touch the air and your body, push outwards and pull inwards. Explore.

- Touch your face and body. Your hands may be drawn to places that need your attention.
- Touch your body as if you were soothing a little child who had been badly frightened. Let your body be moved rather than deciding with your thoughts what you will do.
- When you have explored the upper body, come up on knees, move hips and thighs and finally come to stand and let your arms move, to open, to hug your own body – to dip and sway. Go low, then high. Reach out – stretch and reach outwards, then withdraw and cradle your heart.
- Open your arms and see what that feels like and then wrap your arms around you.

Exploration: Veils and Coloured Scarves

To explore veils as protection.

- Dance, watching the scarf move on the breeze; dance your scarf.
- Wear it as a veil and walk experiencing the air moving the fabric and allowing the air to lift your veil.
- Experience fully what it is like to wear a veil.
- Explore veiling and unveiling.
- If you are dancing with others, do what our DTR dancers did as a goodbye ritual – hold two swathes of light material in the hand of each dancer, hands joined so that you are creating a curtain. Now let another dancer pass through the veil.

Exploration: Touch

To deepen the connection with your own heart and allow that to be extended towards another within respectful boundaries.

- Dance palm to palm with a partner. You can close your eyes or wear a blindfold or, if you prefer, leave your eyes open with a soft focus.

- Breathe. Draw energy through the crown of the head and up from the earth.
- Tune into a soft pink and let the energy run down your arms and into the palms of the other person. The other person closes their eyes and lets you lead.
- He is sensing into his palms where you are leading him. Sense the energy between you. Let your arms move intuitively on the air so you slowly dance his arms and upper body.
- He is sensing into his body, noticing the touch, noticing what it is like for the physical body to be led and the quality of the leading and touching.
- You are staying with the arms and the heaviness or lightness of them.
- Bring the arms upwards in front of his face, moving through the air. Keep it safe though, trust your heart, do not push or be heavy handed.
- Don't push into the other person's energy field. Allow the separateness.
- If the other person is adventurous, you can eventually begin to dance and move around the room. Extending arms, moving closer, playing, all the time keeping your partner safe. You will know this because the arms will be yielding and soft but with a boundary – rather than stiff and heavy. Although of course nothing is wrong.
- Without speaking, swap over.
- As well as playing with leading and following, notice where you lose a sense of your own body and move towards the other and where you can hold your own centre and still be present to the other. Also where you start thinking or spacing out.
- Now experience what it is like to yield and be led. Sometimes the touch is experienced as so tender it has an immediate heart quality. Other times it may be a heavy, swiping or pushing experience.
- If you are not able to stay in your body with someone

touching you, stop them. Wait. You can try again and you can ask for specific touch.
- Practise touch. Touch your body, elbows, knees, heart, flowers, stones, grass, people.
- Breathe and let your breath slow.
- Breathe deeply and easily and touch with reverence.

Exploration: Your Heart Altar
- Play with feathers, wind chimes, clay, massage oil, ribbons, balloons, bubbles, scarves, veils, green things, ivy, soft pink, turquoise, bells, wings, roses, teddies, ice.
- Let your altar come from your own mystery; ask the child within what you need for that altar.
- Put a photograph of yourself as a child there or photographs of your parents as children.

Exploration: Rocking
- Rock your heart as if it were a small baby.
- Use your arms to cradle or let your hands touch the centre of your chest. You could be sitting in a chair or standing.
- Take a moment to pause and rock this child.
- Let your breath become part of that rocking.
- Stay with the rhythm of your heartbeat.

Exploration: Emptying the Heart
- Sit still and centre in on the heart chakra.
- Notice sensation in your chest and upper back.
- Let your hands move gently around your chest, clearing and cleaning.
- Exhale and let your breath and the lightness of air gently clear your heart.
- Breathe in fresh, clean oxygen and light-filled colours.
- Breathe out old stagnant energy.

- Continue until this feels complete and then breathe in the colours again.
- On the out breath, let your voice come and feel it vibrating in your chest.
- Let the heart song be the way you communicate and clear away what needs to be accepted, acknowledged and let go. If words come, then let them be there; they do not have to make sense.
- Be gentle but thorough.
- Let your arms move whatever way they will.
- In your day-to-day practise, notice the sensations in your body when you refer to the past in your mind or when speaking.
- Practise not speaking or thinking about the past at all for one day.

Exploration: Breath/Heart/Rhythm

- How do you rest?
- When you are moving is there a natural contraction and release in your body?
- Does your breath harmonise with this and your heartbeat?
- Is there a rest place in the midst of activity?
- In the ancient art of yoga, every movement harmonises with the next movement. As you move out of bed, practise first breathing and connecting with your heart.
- Now let your body move in harmony with your breath and heart.
- Move fluidly from one movement to another.
- Can you brush your teeth and still stay connected to your heart and breath?
- Let each movement be one of deep rest, resting into the heart and breath.
- Take time during the day to pause, rest, connect with your breath and have a little stretch.

· If you are worried or anxious, take a little time to rock your heart gently.

Exploration: Wishing Well

· Have a heart wishing well – a place you can go to either within or a special place outside under a favourite tree or by a stream. Let this be the place you whisper your heart's wishes, the ones too tender to be spoken loudly.
· Let this be the safe place you whisper your secrets, even the ones you don't know yet.
· You could also make a wishing chair in your house, somewhere you or members of your family can go to sit quietly and not be disturbed and where they can take time to listen to their heart wishes.

Exploration: Balance

· In your movements notice your sense of balance.
· Balance on one leg and let your arms stretch outwards. Then onto the other leg, like a great big bird getting ready to fly.
· Practise balancing on one leg and moving around your room or garden.
· Push your feet into the earth and let your upper body open as you push downwards.
· Let your upper body rotate as you hold your arms open and push your legs rhythmically down into the earth.
· Stand on two legs and come up on your toes, slowly raising your arms and breathing in. As you come down onto your flat feet, breathe out and let your arms move back down to your sides.
· Join your hands together prayer like and slowly begin to move them apart and then gently press them back together.
· Let each movement flow into the other; do not jerk from

one to another. When you are finished, come gently to
rest and allow the movements to inform your body right
through the day.

· Practise this art of surrender by surrendering to your
breath and your true process. Take time to check in with
your heart.

Exploration: Grounding / Balance / Rhythm

· Go onto your right foot, balance – one – then onto left
foot – two – sink feet right down into the earth.

· Notice your balance. 'One and two', and 'one and two',
keeping a nice steady walking rhythm and slowly beginning to raise each foot as you change – almost prancing
like a horse.

· As you move onto one foot, let your upper body move as
well all the time looking for balance.

· Keep doing it until it feels grounded and balanced.

· Then begin hopping on one foot, hold for two, then hop
on the other foot. Again, hold for two.

· When this feels balanced and easy, begin to move around
the room breathing and hopping but not setting 'time
against distance', not trying to achieve anything, simply
noticing the rhythm and your own sense of balance.

· Now let your shoulders and arms come into it, as if you
were a tiger moving through the jungle – let all the muscles be relaxed and sleek, let the mouth open – breathe,
pace your movements – it's a big jungle, no rush.

· 'One-two', on the right and 'one-two', on the left. The
arms and upper body finding a movement that supports
the lower body. If this is paced and grounded enough, you
can go on for hours.

· As you bring in the spirit of the animal, your body can
really begin to embody that spirit and that heart. You can
lift your legs and, as the energy builds around the heart,
you will find yourself having to make sounds, animal

sounds or warrior cries. This is essential to allow the energy to move through the heart. Keeping the same rhythm can be really good for your heart and the movement draws itself around that rhythm and supports it.

· Begin gently at first and build it up over time, it is truly exhilarating.

Exploration: Heart Dance

You can play gentle music for this. We use 'Gabriel's Oboe' from *The Mission*, Ennio Morricone.

· Stand with hands held on your heart. Slowly let one hand slide down until it comes to your side, then the other. Keep your eyes on your hands.
· Bring your right hand forward in front of you and put your right foot behind and left foot forward.
· Slowly raise your hand, stretching arm and hand forward then over your head and backwards in a circular motion (like a wheel) reaching and stretching but without force, eyes on hand all the time, then change hands and feet.
· Now swing your arms forward and backwards. Reaching upwards and downwards. Swinging on your feet as well and gathering momentum as if you were going to take off in flight.
· Gather all that energy in and hold your arms as if you were cradling a baby. Circle to the right then to the left.
· Bend forward to the floor, opening your hands to hand over and surrender your heart's desire, your child, to the earth.
· Rise upwards, opening your arms and chest, pushing your heart forwards, reaching upwards and gathering all the energy from the heavens into your arms.
· Finally, let your hands come back to rest in front of your heart. Rest.
· All the movements are opening, closing, cradling, flying, reaching, stretching.

Exploration: Bird Movements

- See the birds, really see them. Notice their chests and what happens when they sing. Look at nature programmes. I saw a wonderful one on birds of prey, the huge wings moving inwards and outwards – moving the whole bird. The stillness of the wings as the hawk hovers.
- Look at the wings and the breast and copy the movements with your own body. Let your wings open and close, let the energy build, it takes energy to take off, make a 'whoosh' sound like the wings moving through air, feel the movement in your spine, the wings of your back and in your breast.
- Let your legs and knees bend, contract inwards and then hold out the arms, pushing your heart area forward, then sink inwards as the wings close.
- Let your spine be soft and pliable. At times run through the air with your arms outstretched and your heart open. You can feel the air rushing through your chest. Here is really deep learning about balance and rhythm. Fly – rise and sink – hover – soar. Let your breath lead your dance.
- Hold the body like a bird above the earth looking down, balance, then swoop downwards through the space then back upwards again and then hold still before swooping again. Practise this with arms open and then arms by your sides. Feel it in your chest.

Exploration: Left/Right Balance

To explore and strengthen the non-dominant side of the body, releasing creative potential.

- Write with the non-dominant hand. Or paint with both hands. Breathe.
- Let your non-dominant hand lead you.
- Dance, letting the non-dominant side lead you.
- Ask for the movements to come. Let the movement arise from stillness.

- Notice the balance between the right and left side of the body
- Try doing some mirroring exercises, e.g. rotate right hand and arm with body following, catch the movement and repeat with left side, perhaps going in a different direction, then lead with the left and mirror with the right.
- Notice the sensation in the middle of your chest and upper back, check your breathing.

Exploration: Dancing Through the Colours
- Make a body sculpture for each of the colours in your body and psyche. Extend these sculptures into two or three movements for each colour. Move them together to create a rainbow dance.

Exploration: Fingers and Toes
- Lie on the ground and let the tips of your fingers move very gently like the leaves of a tree. Breathe.
- Now bring in your toes, breathe green into the upper chest. Breathe out and let go.
- Notice the tingling sensation.
- When we contract, we can pull energy away from these extremities. Let the tingling sensation move right out to the edges of your leafy fingers and toes.

Exploration: Bubbles and Balloons
- Play the music of the 'Blue Danube'. Dance.
- You could toss a balloon in the air and keep it up there while you dance.
- If you are with others, toss a few balloons up there and blow bubbles and let them burst on the skin.
- Blow bubbles outside and trace a bubble's journey with your eyes.

- Now run after it and see can you burst it.
- Let your voice yell, shriek or laugh.

Exploration: Green Man/Woman

- Think of a man or woman who brings you into your heart or who you perceive to be full of heart or who has a lot of green in the aura. Or a person who seems to be attuned with the air element.
- Today, my inspiration is a woman who has a small healing centre called An Chroí. When she sings she opens her singer's chest with breath and her arms seem to embrace her audience in a wide, sweeping motion. She also rises slightly on her feet as if she were going to fly and her voice soars around the auditorium. All around her are the colours violet, magenta and green.

When we are suffering, when we are separate and hurting, when the arrogance has been beaten out of us, it is this love we long for, the simplicity of tender touch and acceptance. In heart dance we can nurture this quality within our own hearts by dancing with and accepting all the parts of our body, mind and soul, until finally the small will gives up and surrenders. There is often a strong sensation in the heart area, a piercing sensation or a strong throbbing as we are opened from within. I have found that the opening of the heart chakra is a physical reality. Sometimes there is a sensation of bursting open or a strong contraction and release. Sometimes the arms open of their own volition and we expose our heart and chest area in a physical manifestation of that surrender. It is important to be calm and breathe gently. Here is where life itself is entering and thrumming through the small human body and there is a sense of expansion as we endeavour to hold sorrow/pain, release, followed by an authentic, balanced sense of joy and unconditional love experienced in one's own body and emanating outwards to the other bodies around us. There is no will in this, no thought or emotion. We become the rose with a natural scent that permeates the air around us. With grace, that state may come more and more often. For some people it is there all the time and when we fall these people are the ones who extend their hands and their arms and help us to get up.

EXPLORING BLUE – SOUL SONG: CHAKRA 5

Key words or clues: throat, jaw, tongue, teeth, ears, upper arms and thighs, respiratory system.

Fifth chakra	throat – purification (Vissudha-Sanskrit word)
Element	ether
Sense	hearing
Affirmation	'It is safe to hear and speak my truth.'
Colours	blue, madonna blue, sky blue, turquoise
Location	main chakra throat, pharyngeal plexus, associated energy centres related to neck, back of neck, jaw, mouth, teeth, tongue, larynx, ears, nose, lungs, thymus
Endocrine gland	thyroid gland, parathyroid
Secondary chakras	upper arms, thighs
System	respiratory
Clues	sound, song, truth, communication, voice, soul, trust, silence, listening, speaking, vibration, faith, loyalty, grace, integrity, grace, expression, shouting, singing, praising, preaching, protesting, secrets, privacy, discussion, writing, creativity, inspiration, change, communion, conflict, prophet, revolution, rebel, change, resonance, speech
Symbols and props	musical instruments, tuning fork, bell, conche, revolutionary poster, songs, rhymes, blue glass, pens, paints, sacred texts, mandalas, sacred phrases, chants, mudras, forget-me-nots, sky.
Fragrance	myrrh
Food	ice cream, honey, blueberries

Discipline	honesty; creatively expressing truth and inspiration, listening
Imbalances	complaining, lying, criticising, gossip, censorship, control, doubt, prejudice, confusion, talking too much, unable to speak, denial, separation, controlling, frustration/impatience, arguing, under/overactive thyroid, palpitations, sore throats, tonsillitis, creative blocks/addictions, dizziness, tinnitus

I want to sing like birds sing
Not worrying who hears or
What they think

Rumi

We begin with silence and stillness. In the throat chakra, this is particularly important because we are putting more emphasis on sound and listening. The work with sound and colour is so powerful it is essential to add movement so we can embody the voice and the other attributes. These are big clues here: truth, voice, soul, trust, faith and creative expression. In these higher chakras, it is important to slow the movement right down and become very still so that all the systems in the body can resonate with the speed of purification and change. It is imperative not to force the body to make sounds; we are at delicate work here, healing the separation, re-connecting body and soul, body and head. The throat, neck, mouth, jaw and shoulders are areas of huge control and we can hold this area very tightly, clenching the teeth, scrunching the shoulders and pushing the neck and head forwards or backwards. Here our defences are literally fighting for their lives. We work with toning, singing, speaking, storytelling, writing, chanting and the art of listening deeply; listening to our inner truth and finding ways to express this. The throat chakra is the centre of creative expression and we know that we will be working with the saboteur within and our creative blocks, which manifest in the physical body and the throat chakra. The complementary colour is red, and healing in the throat chakra will have a direct effect on the base chakra. It will also influence all the other chakras and energy vibrations in the body. We also work with music and songs from our own and other cultures and simple musical instruments, e.g. tin whistle, bird whistles, singing bowls, bells and sometimes string instruments so we can witness the sound of the string resonating through the body of the instrument.

Around the room as well as the singing bowls and musical instruments we have revolutionary posters, mandalas, sacred words and books, pens and paints, blue lights. We are once again using movement that arises from within.

Music

For dancing the blue, exuberant heart, throat music is good, e.g. lively gospel music that would make you raise your arms and bring down the power. For singing, songs of exile are good, particularly songs or music that bring up a sense of exile within you. Explore those songs and find out about the singer who is singing them. Also songs and music that seem to heal that sense of exile and ones that brings about sensations of safety, comfort and coming home.

· The great singers – John McCormack. Notice what is happening in your body as you listen – people flocked to listen to these people for a reason.
· Harmonic choirs.
· Singing artists: Tim Wheater, *Heartland, Incantation*, www.realmusic.com
· Luka Bloom, *Between the Mountain and the Moon*, 'The Acoustic Motorbike' – exploring the blue, www.lukabloom.com
· Sinead O'Connor, *Universal Mother*, EMI-particularly track 'Thank You'
· Tracey Chapman, 'Talkin bout a Revolution' from her

untitled debut album, Elektra/Asylum Records.
- Tibetan chanting and singing, Sufi-American Indian – prayers and chants from different cultures. Recordings of people using overtone chanting, mouth music. Look for original works.
- Irish *sean-nós* and traditional songs from other cultures, e.g. Romanian women singing.
- Eamon Kelly, *seanchaí* (storyteller)
- Bells, crystal bowls, Tibetan bowls
- Whale sounds

The Colours Around You - Blue

Blue is one of the greatest antiseptics in the world. It is also known as the healing colour. It cools and calms us and also brings about a state of expansion. Looking up at a blue sky we can feel this expansion. A blue light is comforting if you have a temperature. It affects the throat centre and the thyroid gland. It calms the whole system and is good for any throat condition or itchy hot rashes. It is often used as a protective colour for example: Mary's mantle of blue. The colour blue is associated with hope, faith, trust, devotion, inspiration, loyalty and integrity. Too much blue can make us withdrawn so we need to use it with a warm colour – orange or rose pink. Royal blue brings us into our spiritual authority. Use it with peach, yellow, orange or rose pink. Royal blue clears our perceptions so they become more finely tuned. Turquoise calms the nervous system and is used in burn units in hospitals as it is good for shock and for burning sensations. Aqua and turquoise are two of the most healing colours we need at this time. They open us up to new truths coming in, and towards a more honest way of living and being. They are particularly good in a therapy room or an artist's, singer's or writer's studio – combine with peach or a little orange. These colours are good in children's rooms. For small babies leave the colours pale and pastel and add pink or lavender on different walls all toning into each other. The colour turquoise is related to the thymus gland where an eighth chakra is said to be forming from one of the minor chakras there. Most people doing our work have certainly felt a lot of sensation in this area. As this chakra opens and flowers it brings together heart and throat chakras. This area of the body ages and stiffens prematurely in the western body. Breathing turquoise into this area helps to soften and rejuvenate the area, strengthens the immune system and helps us with our communication. It is particularly helpful for fears about public speaking. Use turquoise if you are nervous. It also helps us in any artistic project or giving workshops, performances, or talks and helps us to communicate more clearly in intimate relationships. It is a very good colour when we need to bring our inspiration to the earth and give it a voice – because it is working with the heart and throat it helps the voice to embody. A turquoise wrap is wonderful protection or wear turquoise in a necklace, earrings, scarf or tie. Turquoise and certain aqua greens are beautiful colours used in combination. Just think of the warm seas. Use turquoise and aqua with a coral pink for deep healing of the resonant voice.

Exploration: Jaw and Mouth

- Close your eyes for a moment and scan your body.
- Notice the energy around your jaw, mouth, neck, throat and shoulders.
- Gently begin to open and close your mouth, very relaxed and slow.
- Breathe in and out through your mouth and nose and see if you can synchronise the opening and closing of your mouth with the breath.
- Relax the jaw, face, eyes, scalp. Let the tension begin to seep out through the pores of the skin and on the breath.
- Bring in yawning and a little groaning low down in the body.
- See if you can bring that groaning down into achy, stiff or constricted places in your body. See if you can massage these areas with your groans and moans.

· Beginning with your fingers, allow your body to move sensually – groaning, moaning and yawning.
· Stretch the muscles in your upper back, shoulders and upper arms as you groan, moan, yawn and open your mouth wide.

Exploration: Listening
· Pause for a moment and listen.
· When your thoughts come in, gently turn them down and listen to the sounds in your body, in your room, outside the room, in the air.
· Are you aware of all the sounds you filter out as a matter of course?
· How often do you notice birdsong or the sweetness of a baby's voice or the sound of water or fire?
· Do you ever allow yourself really to listen to all the sounds in your house?

Exploration: Gibberish
· Don't use words, just babble gibberish. Give out, argue, hold forth. Babble loud, low, up high, in an excited voice, in a monotone, deep and low.
· Make faces, let your tongue go wild. Now laugh: a big, high posh lady's laugh, a big belly laugh, every type of a laugh you can make. Let these laughs come from different parts of your body.
· For example, the high posh lady's laugh will be up around the neck and chest and you might find yourself putting your hands there in a prissy way, whereas a big dirty laugh will come from lower down in the belly and there can be an impulse to slap someone's back, like a crowd in the pub after a match.
· This is great fun if you do it with a group of people as the laughter has a way of taking off. You could try pointing at people and laughing at them and notice where that laugh

is in the body. Don't censor yourself; make every type of
sound that you can.

Exploration: Voices

·   Do you notice the false note in your own voice?
·   Do you feel you speak in a monotone sometimes? What
    kind of situation makes you speak in a monotone?
·   Do you notice if your voice gets high and ungrounded?
·   Do you ever notice when your voice is varied and expressive?
·   Do you ever hear, feel and enjoy your own voice sounds?
·   Do you notice other people's voices?
·   Do you find it hard to listen to people talking sometimes?
·   Do you notice what element in their speech turns you off?
·   Do you ever listen to the breath and how it is used when
    the person is speaking?
·   Do you take the time to be still and listen?

Exploration: Complaining

·   How often do you complain? Do you complain directly
    to the person who is annoying you or do you complain
    generally to others about situations that annoy you?
·   Do you often praise others? Do you often criticise?
·   In conversation, do you tend to generalise or do you speak
    personally?
·   Do you argue a lot? Do you enjoy discussion or debate?
·   Do you tend to agree and back off when someone argues?
·   Do you want to prove, to explain, to give information or
    advice?

Exploration: Expansive Movement

·   If you notice yourself or others moving, you will begin
    to notice how constricted the movements can be. Rarely
    would you see someone putting their hands up into the

air above their heads. Sometimes a preacher will use this gesture or football fans at a match, but for most people it is as if a line has been drawn that they cannot cross over. Each person has a comfort zone and as we get older that comfort zone can constrict even more.

· Begin to expand your range of movement options. Raise your hands up high, reach as high as you can and gaze upwards at the sky. Move up into the blues and violets. Move your arms and hands around and feel the air above your head and all the currents of energy above your body.

· Sometimes your movements will be airy and light. Experiment with pushing the air as if it were more solid and feel that push in your arms and upper body, feel the stretch in the middle of your body as you push your feet and legs down into the ground.

· Now move down to your heart, then solar plexus level, midway between earth and sky, and see what kind of movements you can make here. Can you put out your leg into this space, your body parallel to the ground? Explore the space all around your body in whatever way you can, all the time breathing and moving sensually. Don't push your body, but do challenge yourself a little.

· Sink down to earth now and explore the movements you can make low down to the ground. Once again, explore the space and the ground around you.

· Rise and then sink again. What part of your body is leading? Can you let your elbow lead you down to the ground? Perhaps your chest could lead you up off the ground.

· Can you explore twisting your arms into different shapes and your body into different shapes?

· Imagine that you are standing in a cube. See what it would be like to place one part of your body in one corner and let another part reach towards another corner. Play with this using opposite corners and being aware of three levels within the cube.

· By expanding your movement range, you are beginning to

revolutionise your whole way of being. Take possession of space that you have not occupied before. If you have never explored the space behind your back, then what's there?

· Move out into the space around your body; move into the circle around your body, the cube around your body or the triangle.

· As you have worked with the explorations in the previous chakras, you have begun to embody more fully on the earth and you have become more and more aware of your inner space and your kinaesthetic sense of movement, even the most subtle movements within your own body. Because of this you can now begin to move that energy out into the space around you without dissociating or becoming overly identified with what is outside your own system.

· Move out into the space around you now and draw it back into your body. Play with your internal space and your external space letting movements rise from within and move outwards and then letting movements begin way out in the space around you and drawing the movement back into the core of your body.

· Advance and retreat, move from one side to another. Move lightly and airily and then explore moving in an earthy way or with fire movements. Let different parts of your body lead you. If you are in a big, uncluttered space like your garden, explore advancing and retreating a little faster than is comfortable for you. Rise and sink. Notice the sensations in your body as you do this. These movements can give rise to feelings of exhilaration and expansiveness or you may feel dizzy or uncomfortable, or unexpected feelings of sadness or anger may emerge. Don't push through these feelings, slow the movements down and take time to dance these feelings and explore them fully.

Exploration: Make a Revolutionary Speech

· Hold your arms open and above your head. Open your mouth and make a speech, even if the speech is in gibberish, or take something you feel strongly about and write and make a speech about it.

· Notice the sensations in your body, notice where the energy goes and moves. Really go for it – shout at them, gesticulate, rally them forward and rouse them out of their apathy.

· Notice if you get spacey or feel ungrounded. Open out your legs and plug into the earth with your feet.

Exploration: Inner Conflict

· Begin to notice conflicting creative impulses, for example two of mine are a) a fascination with finding a home and settling down; and b) the urge to take to the road and travel like a gypsy. Between these two extremes lies a wealth of creativity. If I decide that one way is the right way and try to eradicate the other part of me, this part will go into shadow and I will act it out in destructive ways. Whereas if we can hold the two impulses within, they can spark each other creatively. Be on the look-out for these apparent contradictions in your own life.

· Now take time to dance these two impulses. Notice where they are originating from in your body and take time to explore this fully. For example, when I tune into my settling down, homey movements, I find myself hugging and caressing my upper arms and kind of snuggling down into my body. I notice that my eyes close and I make little contented, purring noises. When I tune into my gypsy traveller, I begin to look around and stretch my body like a cat. I also notice that I am licking my lips and making little excited sounds. Somewhere in there as well is a sensation in the solar plexus and as I actually go as far as planning to pack, my body contracts and my ankles and feet stiffen up and I notice that I am beginning to hold them quite rigidly. As

I begin to dance all these apparent conflicting sensations within my own body, they come into communication with each other. What is going on in my feet and ankles that somehow relates to this feeling in my solar plexus? What is all that pleasure about when I stretch like a cat?

· Take time to move to your own apparent conflicts within your own body.

· Find music that supports them.

· There may not be an immediate resolution. Do not look for this or any other kind of *result*. You are simply listening, so all of these different ways of being are experienced, witnessed and, if you need to, you can let the different voices emerge. You do not need to use words; let sounds express the sensations.

Exploration: Shout

· Do you feel you have to shout to be heard? Do you ever shout and scream?

· In what ways do you censor yourself? How do you let others censor you?

· Practise shouting, not to oppress or bully anyone but simply to hear yourself shout and experience what that is like in your body. Be careful to stay grounded and playful. Be careful not to go into a spacey screaming and leave your body. Stay grounded and don't constrict your voice in your neck.

Exploration: Let the Gossip Write

· Let your gossip voice go wild. Be as bitchy as you can be. Gossip about this person and that – use gibberish if you like.

· See where the gossip is resonating in your body.

· Notice what it is like to sit down with someone intimately and have a good old gossip – the lovely false power as you trade opinions about someone who is not there.

- Notice when you are enjoying it and when it feels a bit uncomfortable.
- See now if the character you are describing could be turned into a fictional character. The things you are honing in on and the way you are embellishing them are all ways to tap into your own creativity.

Exploration: Whispering

- Whisper. You do not have to use words; whisper the sensations in your body. Let the whispering find the words. Let those hidden parts of you whisper to you and you can confide and whisper back. Whisper to trees, to rivers, to your pillow – your invisible friend.
- Draw a circle on a large piece of paper. This can be your sacred circle. Within this circle you can write things that you would never dare to say. Then you can veil or decorate these whispers with lovely coloured crêpe paper or little gold designs. You can put paintings in there or symbols. Now place this sacred circle on your blue altar.

Exploration: Blue

- Breathe blue into the throat area and all around your upper body. Then let this colour move down through your body, through your veins.
- Stretch out your arms. Let your mouth open and allow sound to come through your wide mouth, being careful to leave your throat relaxed and open.
- Begin to make different shapes with your mouth, sending the sound up into the roof of your mouth or into the cavern of your skull then way down low into your belly. Let your voice lead you.
- Move your arms and hands and move the blue light around your body.
- Keep your body grounded – tail, hands and feet.

Exploration: Listening to Your Voice and the Sounds Around You

- Listen to your voice when you are speaking. Notice the pitch and tone, the false note, the deep trembling one.
- Notice your voice making strange sounds, wobbling, trembling, rasping. Let it be and simply listen.
- When you speak, can you feel the connection between your voice, throat and heart? Is your voice coming from within your body?
- Does your body feel connected to your voice and what you are saying? Just notice, do not judge because it takes time to find your own voice.
- Practise listening with your full body and with all of your senses. Let the sounds come in through the pores of your skin.
- Listen and then let your ears expand as if you could turn a dial and tune into sounds further outside your immediate environment. Go right into the tree with the bird. Fly beside that swan and listen to her wings moving through the air. Sit in the car with that passing driver.
- Because of the noise in our world or the voices shouting in our heads or the people who have actually shouted at us, we have numbed out our full potential for listening. Put in space in your day, even only a minute, when you can allow yourself to hear more fully. Notice the swirls of sound, the vibration of sound and the tones that lie just underneath the sound.
- When you are listening, notice where you are listening from; is it your ears or does your throat seem to be picking up on the transmission of sound? Are you breathing? Is the sound coming to you through the air? Are your thoughts tuning out certain sounds? Don't resist or block some sounds while allowing others in.
- When you have listened, let your own voice find its place within all of these sounds. Find a way to harmonise and play with the birdsong or the sound of the trees swishing in the wind or the tapping of the keyboard of a computer

or typewriter or the sounds in your car. See if you can connect and touch the birdsong with your own voice. See if you can send your sound to the tree while it is still resonating within your own body.

· When you have finished, become aware of your other senses, your sense of smell, taste or touch. Do colours seem brighter?

Exploration: Sounding

· Make sounds – percussive sounds 'Ca Ba Ga'. Make them sharp and sudden. Let the solar plexus move to expel these sounds

· Then make more floating sounds, 'Bluuuuuuuuuuuuuuu – eeeeeeeeeee – aaaaaaaaaaaaa – uuuuuuuuuuu – ooooooooo'. Once again, bring these sounds from the tummy. Also draw the sounds down into the body.

· Move your mouth: with 'la la la – da dad a da – mama-mama'; then, 'MMMMMMMMM', going up into the head vibrating the lips and humming like a bee; then 'SSSSSSSSSSSSSSS' like a snake. Then big 'HAAAAAAA' from the chest. Make nasal sounds as if you had a cold. Feel the sound vibrate in the area around the nose and forehead.

· Experiment – make other sounds and move your face. Make silly faces and sounds down deep in your body and then way up high and all the places in middle.

Exploration: the Energetic Voice

· Become more aware of how you are using the energy coming through your voice.

· Notice when you become tired or when the energy seems to die in a conversation. Notice if you try to keep the conversation going and what that costs you energetically.

· If you are suppressing your voice, once again begin to notice how that feels; do you become tired or lose energy?

- Use colours to draw or paint the energy coming through your body, the lungs, the larynx and out of the mouth; are there places where it is stuck or blocked?
- Add words or symbols to represent where this energy is going.
- If you are a real talker, practise not talking so much. Hold the silence and allow others to speak. Use that energy to write, paint, make a collage or knit a jumper. Use that energy to sound, chant or sing songs.
- If you find it difficult to talk, then use the suppressed energy to do any of the above but particularly chanting and sounding.

Exploration: Practise Silence

- Take an hour or even a day or longer to be silent. Eat meals in silence or take a walk with someone else in silence.
- Take a day of not reading, listening to the radio or watching TV. Switch off the phone and mobile phone and don't text.
- When you are driving, do not listen to music; listen instead to the sound of the car and the sounds outside of the car.
- Sometimes we can be silent with our voices, but our thoughts are babbling away and our energy is chaotic. Find ways to still the mind. One of the most useful ways is to go around the body allowing each part of it to relax completely. When the body relaxes and lets go, the thinking stops.

Exploration: Energy Focus

- Make a list of tasks you need to do each morning. Don't say you have no time; believe me, this will save you so much time and it will also save you from expending your energy needlessly.
- Become still and ask for help to focus on what you need to do that day to fulfil your creative potential, to honour your

soul path; use whatever words seem appropriate to you. If you are addicted to taking care of other people, it might simply be to ask for help to mind your own business.

- Sometimes people say to me, well it is obvious what I have to do, I need to get up and feed my baby. This may very well be your creative and soul path and of course that is a need, not a desire. You need to feed your baby. However when your baby is asleep, what do you do? Perhaps it might be good to take a walk with your baby in that place that inspires you. I remember getting little intuitive messages to pick up the phone and ring someone or go and visit them only to find that my day was filled with riches instead of routine.

- Sit in silence. Listen and be still for a moment, now look at your list. I always add the words 'something else' in case there is something I have not thought of. You can use a pendulum or you can simply run your finger along the list and see where your finger vibrates slightly, or it might be that your eye falls on one sentence, e.g. 'go and buy those paints' or, 'ring and make that appointment with that therapist' or, 'deal with that money worry, it's interfering with my peace of mind'. It will not necessarily feel like the comfortable option, but deep down in your tummy you know it's the one.

- Now move down your list and ask for priority two, three, and so on. Researchers into business practice say that if you prioritise and do the first two things on your list, you are operating at something like 80% of your potential. Isn't that comforting?

- At the end of the day you can look back on your list. How much energy did you expend on the different projects or tasks? How much energy did you receive back? How do you feel now that you finally bought those paints, made that appointment, had that walk?

- The next day do it again. I usually write about my dreams and how I am feeling first, then sit in meditation and use my voice or some gentle movement. Others dance first thing or practise yoga. Then I make my list.

Exploration: Humming

· Dance slowly and, as you dance, hum. It does not have to be a particular tune, simply let your voice hum and follow the hum through your body.

· If the hum is rising and going high, let your body rise. If the voice is low, let your body sink and move downwards. Jiggly hums get little jiggly movements.

· Play with this yourself. Then let your voice go high and your body low and vice versa.

Exploration: Toning Through the Chakras

· Lie down flat, with a flat cushion underneath your head so that your chin is well tucked in and the back of the neck extended. If your back is uncomfortable, raise your knees.

· Breathe in colour to the base then breathe the colour out into the air. Go through each of the chakras – breathe in colours and breathe out. Fill your energy field with the bright, natural colours.

· When you are ready, begin to let your voice come by resting it on your breath. You are keeping 50 percent of your voice inside your body and letting 50 percent float on the air outside your skin.

· Breathe in and let your voice rest on the colour. Let the colours come intuitively – the red may change to pink or magenta. Let your voice slide between the chakras. You might find yourself resisting certain colours, for example you might reject a dark green then ask your intuition to guide you towards a green that you need. Sometimes we reject the very colours that we need, so if you need a green and cannot tolerate the colour, look in nature for something you can relate to, perhaps the colour of moss or the greens in the sea. Find a colour you feel comfortable with.

· Move up through the body and back down again. Let your voice be deep and go higher as you travel through the instrument of your body. Let your voice make strange noises or glitches.

· Be careful not to force sound in the throat or you will damage the larynx – let the throat be as open as a cave and send your voice down deeply into your body.

· When you are toning the third eye, let your voice come from there and resonate through the nose and skull. A bit like you have a cold.

· Practise this and listen to voices chanting from different cultures and see if you can bring your voice from the same part of your body. Always be gentle and let your voice lead you. It may come strongly at times, at other times faintly. Trust your voice

· Notice what sounds come from the different chakras. For example, a voice giving out the news would probably come from the solar plexus. Antoinette says that Marilyn Monroe singing 'Do it Again' comes sweetly from the sacral centre. Martin Luther King's voice seems to vibrate through all the chakras. If you were holding a little baby and patting its back, the sound 'ahhh, ahhhh' would probably come through your heart and throat, connecting them up in a gentle easy way. Middle Eastern chants come from the bellows of the body and echo in the third eye. As you listen to different people singing, notice where there voice is resonating in your body.

· If you practise this enough, you will eventually be able to bring your voice at will from the different chakras. Realise how powerful this is; if you are in the midst of people arguing you could bring your voice from your heart and have a profound effect on the group.

· If you do develop this power, then it is in your own interests to use it wisely. It is also important to realise that your voice does have power and to be aware of what you are saying. Your words have power. Speak well of other people or not at all. Speak in a loving way about yourself. Speak positively about your life and life direction.

- In conflict situations, once again realise that your voice has more power if you can bring it from your heart and speak lovingly about the conflict. Attack always brings counter attack and returns swiftly to your own body. Speak to others as you would have them speak to you. For in truth you are speaking to yourself.

Exploration: Once Upon a Time

- Begin 'once upon a time there was a little girl/boy and he liked the colour ...'
- Pick a situation in your life that has had or is having a strong impression on you; a moment in time when your life changed or you saw things differently. Tell the story to someone, or to your teddy, to a tree, or to your dog. Let the words come; even if they are stumbling at first, you will find your way.
- Find stories that you loved as a child and read them again or get someone to read one to you.
- Start a storytelling group – exaggeration is allowed and it does not all have to be true or rather it could be 'made-up truth', Bernard McLaverty's words in a writing workshop.
- Picture your life as a film. Pick a certain time in your life. Who is playing you? what actors are playing other key people in your life? At what moment does the film begin? At what moment in the film do you come forward in your seat and begin to cheer on the heroine? Where does it end? What music would be your theme music or what other music would you play through the film and at what stages?

Exploration: Your Blue Energy

· Draw a quick sketch of your mouth, jaw, larynx, neck and lungs. It need only be understandable to you.

· Using colours, draw the energy spiralling up through your lungs and out of your mouth.

· How are you using this energy? Can you contain the momentum of creative energy or do you dissipate it by talking, texting, emailing, phoning? Write in words around your sketch.

· Look energetically at the story of Dracula and the vampires. Do you feed people with the energy in your throat? Do you feed off them? For example, do you keep asking questions just to be around a certain person? Do you keep speaking for the sake of staying with someone or keeping their attention when the energy has died and it is time to go?

· Do you ever notice that you could feel completely down but after speaking with a particular person you feel full of energy and know it's because you have been nourished and fed by their energy? Do you acknowledge that to them and exchange energy in some way, buying them dinner or sending flowers?

· Do you ever notice that after speaking to certain people you feel drained and exhausted?

· Sometimes old grief or feelings may have been triggered by a certain conversation, but sometimes we are using our voices to feed off each other in ways that ultimately dissipate our energy. When the energy is with us, we are using universal energy and both people are uplifted by the exchange. There is a different sensation and feeling quality to the conversation. There is an equal exchange and good boundaries are in place. You will not feel drained or uneasy after the exchange. You will not feel guilty or resentful.

Exploration: Your Songs

- Do you remember the songs you sang as a child? Or the first record you bought? The songs you bothered to learn?
- Can you remember old advertisement jingles, nursery rhymes, skipping rhymes?
- What songs did your parents or grandparents sing? Did they sing? Or hum or whistle? What kind of music did they like?
- When you are remembering, don't just recall, sing the songs.

Exploration: Back to Back Massage

- Ask someone to play this game with you. If there is no one, then sit with your back against a cushion supported by the wall. With a partner sit with backs touching as much of the surface of the back as you can or the cushion.
- Now you begin to tone then sing; lines of songs, lullabies, rhymes or anything else that comes to you. You are attempting to massage the other person's back or the cushion with your voice. Try not to become self-conscious; the aim is to massage the other person's back not to sing well. This will bring your voice right down into your body and resonating through your bones, muscles and organs.

Exploration: Making Music

- Listen to voices that sound true and original, singers who seem to sing their truth and singers who inspire you with their stories. Listen to them live when you can.
- Most of all, sing yourself – hum, chant, sing – make music with your own voice or with simple instruments, e.g. a tambourine or a bird whistle. Find a group of people to sing and play music with in a simple, easy way.
- Note down songs that you love and singers you were drawn to through your life. Spend time in world music shops. Learn songs, sing them and deepen the vibration of the song with your toning practise.

· We highly recommend going to music-lover friends and asking them to play their favourite music for you. They will love that and you will be educated about their music and about them. When a song stirs you, ask – where in my body does this song or piece of music resonate?

Exploration: Singing the Wisdom

· When you use your voice, be conscious of the energy you call upon. If you use ancient chants and words, you are calling on the energy of that particular wisdom tradition. For example, if you are calling on the name Jesus Christ, this is a very powerful name. However, you are also calling up energy associations you or others have with the name including the abuses carried out in this name. Therefore, be very clear about how you are using your voice. For example, if you are chanting make the intention to call on the pure and original energy associated with this name. When we called on the myth 'The Children Of Lir', we were using it like magic to call up the wisdom held in the words and in the story. When we called on the healing of the swan, we called on the pure energy that comes through the swan.

· You can use your own sounds to call up and connect with airwaves you would like to tune into. For example, if you wanted to enhance your natural healing abilities you could connect with the purest form of the hands-on healer. Use your voice to connect with this vibration but if you find that this does not resonate with you, simply use your voice to call on the vibration you need or the colour and the rest will emerge mysteriously. Because, just as you have learned to listen, know that you are being listened to.

Communion

Bathing in blue waters and painting blue opens up the soul–body connection. This colour opens us up to an ethereal stillness that is the beginning of communication with the soul, sometimes the beginning of a psychic opening, and then we pass through this to the pure stillness where there is no thought only communion with that stillness that seems to be nothing. This is the deepest communion in the throat chakra and it goes below all words, thoughts or seeing. If we could not speak, hear or see, still this communion exists. It resides in our cells and in the breath that breathes life into us. Exploring the blue eventually, softly, surely brings us home and there is nothing to say now, for in this place all is known.

Exploring Indigo – Trance Dance: Chakra 6

Key words or clues: forehead, brow, eyes, lower head, pituitary gland, movements are reflective, inward moving.

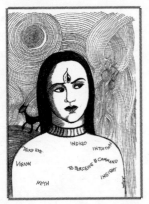

Sixth chakra	third eye – to perceive and command
Element	light
Sense	clairvoyance
Endocrine gland	pituitary
Affirmation	'I am prepared to see this differently', 'I draw back all projections and look within'
Colours	indigo lavender/pink, magenta, silvery dawn/dusk
Location	forehead, brow, related to eyes, sinuses, lower head
Clues	intuition, vision, quest, initiation, illusion, seer/teacher/shaman, inward looking, oracle, discernment, myth, image, changing forms, signs, patterns, omens, metamorphoses, conjuring, midnight, twilight, superstition, insight, imagination, aspiration, mandalas, ghosts, fears, projections, confusion/clarity, illusion, curse, vow, discipline, frequencies/wavelengths, focus, bliss
Symbols and props	white cloth, ink, candle, lantern, robes, bindy (Indian symbol placed on 3rd eye area), sacred ritual/initiation, ceremonial props, feathers, rattle, smudge stick, (Native American cedarwood and sage to clear the atmosphere) sacred oil, holy water, chalice, oracle aids, crystal ball, I Ching, tarot/divining cards, runes, pendulum, aura soma,

	prisms, aura glasses, pinhole glasses, dreams, symbols, astrological chart
Fragrance	frankincense, myrrh, sage, cedarwood
Food	blackberries, aubergines, plums, grapes, wine
Discipline	responsibility for own actions, thoughts and perceived reality, perceiving habitual patterns, energy, karma, signs, seeing through illusions, conditioning, projections and personal opinions, disciplining thoughts and whole system, discernment, wisdom, respect, containment
Imbalances	delusions, confusion, denial, loss of autonomy, superstition, fear of unfamiliar, curses, phobias, depression, vision problems, tunnel vision, headaches (thumping, raging), sinusitis, insomnia, inability to focus; lack of imagination and creativity; being drawn into other people's stories, projections, fantasies and so on

All Indians must dance, everywhere, keep on dancing. Pretty soon in next spring Great Spirit come.

Wovoka, The Paiute Messiah,
extract from *The Ghost Dance*

As we enter the indigo light, we become silent; we hold the energy and do not dissipate it with chatter. This is a holy place. We are on sacred ground. Life is going to intimate to us what it needs from us. Everywhere there will be signs.

We begin now to enter the higher tones, or the more nasal chants, the music that cries out to God. We use ritual music from every culture. In every culture there are sacred ways to still the mind: trance dancing, drumming, meditation, tantric lovemaking, yoga and other movement disciplines, divination aids, astrology, sacred art. In all of these disciplines, the thinker must learn to serve a higher purpose. Within the indigo ray, we meet the inner teacher, the seer, the mystic, moving below and, beyond what we think we know, we ask for the humility to follow our sacred dreams and fulfil our destiny.

The word indigo conjures up eastern adventures, myths and stories of old, magic lamps and dark caves that turn into treasure troves. The rich indigos, magentas and violets in the aura intimate great spiritual power and knowing that comes with age, experience that is only possible in a life fully lived.

As we move in the indigo light, once again we may notice that the room seems colder. There is a fear here that is different than the fight-or-flight fear in earth dance or the fear of the mind in fire dance; this is an ancient superstitious fear that makes the hairs stand up at the back of your neck. It is the fear of the banshee or of the grim reaper, death, ghost stories, stories of fairies who exchange a child for one of their own, a changeling. Fear of seeing our shadow selves, fear of God or what we perceive God to be – a judging man with a big white beard who will make you pay for your sins and who sees your guilt. Fear of the devil and what we perceive the devil to be. Our issues around formal religion and religious abuse rise up so we can see them clearly. Dancers often find that old fears of the psychic, the gypsy, the shaman or the witch rise up in them or a fear of being seen as one of these and being tortured or killed. We may feel strong connections with animals, wolf magic, cat magic and the companionship of the familiar. There is also the fear of seeing past what everyone accepts as normal. Sometimes dancers feel uncomfortable with formal ritual or ceremony because this power has been abused in the past. As we dance in this indigo light, these issues rise up to be transformed and healed and we reclaim the power of ritual, sacred art, initiation and ceremony as a way to celebrate, create and heal our own lives.

Music

- Sacred Spirit (mentioned in fire dance)
- Robbie Robertson, *Music for the Naïve American*, Capitol Records, 'The Ghost Dance' and other tracks.
- Recordings of prayers, chants and songs from other cultures bring us into the energy of the third eye
- *The Whirling Dervishes of Damascus*, *Le Chant Du Monde*, Ensemble Al-Kindi, Sheikh Hamza Shakkur
- Shamanic drumming
- Drums, rattles, voice, chanting
- Lisa Gerrard, *The Mirror Pool*, Warner Brothers records
- Seán Davies – 'The Deer's Cry' from the album *The Pilgrim*, Tara Music

The Colours Around You – Indigo

Indigo touches our deep inner fears and helps to release them. It is a powerful painkiller and is good for headaches, insomnia, sinusitis, tinnitus, deafness and eye-strain. It affects the skeleton and is a great purifier of the blood stream. It depresses the nerves and lymphatics. It is also good for rheumatism and arthritis, varicose veins, insomnia and bruising. Because it heals the etheric body, it can remove pain but pain is a warning sign so always get qualified advice. Breathe it in, or use stained glass and receive it through the light. Wear it or put a coloured cloth near your bed or an indigo pillow slip for insomnia.

The darkness of indigo can bring up a lot of our fears so use sparingly and not at all if it is having a strong effect. For strong emotional states, consult a colour therapist. Use indigo with pink. Pink calms the emotions and the muscular system. Indigo, with its complementary colour orange or orange/gold, is extremely powerful. I find these two colours, particularly orange on the deep indigo, bring a deep sense of joy, calm and well-being for me. They are a good balance but once again only use intuitively and these colours would not be good in your house. Instead use blues and oranges. Royal blue brings out loyalty and integrity, but again use sparingly. When we are making our third eye altar, we often use indigo and white with a little pink and violet heather. We also use a gold or white candle. Sometimes we put a candle onto a mirror. Once again this whole effect can be softened with the use of pink or lavender and the complementary orange on a light box or candle. Working the indigo ray you may find you are falling asleep or in an altered state, so bring in the warmer colours to balance. The indigo ray is one of stillness. Give yourself time to be still.

Exploration: Living the Vision
· Pause for a moment.
· Are you feeling stuck in your life?
· What do you need to give up so that you have more energy to move forward?
· The first thing that comes into your mind's eye – that is the one that is dissipating your energy.

Exploration: Connecting with the Intelligence and Power in Nature
· Make time to go on a walk in a natural place that has strong medicine for you. A sacred site or a grove of trees.
· Let go of your everyday concerns and before you enter this place ask the intelligence in nature for permission to enter.
· Move into the aura or energy here consciously. Be conscious of the trees or mountains or sea or river looking at you as you arrive.
· Make an offering to the nature spirits of this place.
· Give thanks and then let yourself be drawn to a place to sit or lie.
· Now simply receive the energy and beauty.
· Allow your eyes to trace the leaves or the shape of a stone or branch.
· Wait and breathe.
· You may find that a sound courses through your body, or a cry

or a sob, a shudder or simply a sense of well-being and peace.
- Or you may find that you cannot still your thoughts. Practise by telling your thoughts to the tree or the river until your mind quietens.

Exploration: Trance Dance

- Warm up through the other chakras.
- Use music or sacred chant such as Nuzrat Fat ali Khan. Shamanic drumming is good and Sufi music from the whirling dervishes is good, as is Native American music, Irish *sean-nós* or prayers from different cultures.
- Keep the steps simple, with a simple rhythm. Soften your eyes and let the lids half close, use your peripheral vision. Keep a good rhythm.
- African tribes use a simple toe-to-heel slide, the spine supple like a snake. It is the same in Irish *sean-nós* – a simple toe-to-heel slide and the beat of the *bodhrán* is our way to the wild mind.
- Choose one simple step, engaging your whole body and letting your head bob gently on the top of your spine.
- Keep the body soft and fluid; don't jar your body. Begin to elaborate on this simple movement, bringing in your shoulders and chest. Move forwards and backwards and from side to side.
- Find a way to repeat this step so your whole body is engaged in a simple repetitive rhythm.
- Go with the energy in your own body. If you become tired and heavy, don't stop; dance the heaviness. Sometimes it can feel like you are dancing through sludge, then the energy will change and lighten. Sometimes the energy will speed up and you will feel invigorated as the energy moves up through your legs and grounds down through your body and into the earth.
- Practise this way of dancing. In tribal communities these meditative dances can go on for hours and days and the

dancing healers receive many messages that they pass onto the tribe. Obviously you need to build up to this. Go at your own pace, do not force or try to achieve.

· Eventually let the dance slow to its own ending.

· In the stillness afterwards, rest, listen and see with your inner eye.

· Ask a question relevant to your life right now; make the question as clear and concise as possible. Ask to be guided intuitively and through your dreams.

Exploration: Dissolving the Barriers

· Examine any barriers that prevent you moving forward with your vision.

· Write about this barrier as fully as you can.

· Dance it and notice where you can feel it in your body.

· Sound it and once again see where you can feel this barrier in your body and voice.

· In what chakra do you think this barrier is? Perhaps it seems to reside in more than one.

· At this point you may wish to bring in the exercise on expanding your vision on page (see below)

· You can now say, 'Please help me to see this differently. Please help me to dissolve the barriers in my own mind that prevent me from serving you with all the gifts and talents you have given me.'

Exploration: Expand Your Vision

· Stand looking ahead. Bring your straight arm upwards so that your hand is at eye level.

· Keeping your hand in your field of vision, move your hand to the right, following with your eyes but keeping your head still. Stop before your hand leaves your field of vision.

· Now follow your hand back to the front. Breathe consciously while you are doing this, keeping your awareness on what you are doing.

- Now do this with the other hand and then both hands together – one going to right and one to left.
- Close your eyes and feel the effects of this exercise in your body.
- Notice your vision afterwards.
- Peripheral vision is your complete field of vision. In life we forget to look around up – down – left – right. Expand your vision and, as you dance, notice what ways your eyes move as you move.
- Which moves first – your eyes or your body?
- Practise softening your eyes. Notice when the energy jumps our through your eyes projecting outwards at a passing woman or man or some writing/image.
- Let your eyes rest peacefully in their sockets. Receive with your eyes instead of projecting outwards. Receive the nature and beauty around you.
- Notice other people's eyes. Watch the way the energy seems to come out of the eyes sometimes, particularly when people are watching television or at the computer.
- Trace the outline of objects with your eyes. Notice if you stop breathing. In this way you relax the eye muscles.
- Trace the outline of something that is far away from you and then something quite near.

Exploration: the Mirrors of the Soul

- Look at photographs of people from earth-based cultures or cultures where there are receptive water qualities, for example, India.
- Notice the receptive quality in the eyes.
- Become aware of the muscles of your eyes and the connection to your breath.
- Notice when your eyes become fixed or the fixed frown on your forehead.

· Don't change it, simply observe.
· Are you breathing?
· What are you thinking?
· Have you blocked out the present moment?
· Are you aware of your surroundings, the people around you?
· What are you fixating on?

Exploration: Pause

· Sit in silence and observe thoughts moving across your mind.
· Do not follow them as they jump from one to another; hold the pause between the thoughts for as long as is comfortable.
· Look at your thoughts, but stay detached from them.
· When you are ready, begin to dance to the silence between the thoughts. This may be a very gentle dance just with your fingers or arms. Notice the thought coming and then dance again in the silence.
· During the day whenever you feel fear or your body is stiffening up, or your eyes are tense, pause, focus on your thoughts, detach gently, make one simple gesture, raise your hand and follow it with your eyes or join your hands and raise them to your third eye, then your lips.

Exploration: Seeing Clearly

· When you sit to meditate, notice if you cannot be still. Are there aches or pains or vague feelings of anxiety that are preventing your body being still in your meditation and in your life?
· Ask to see what situation in your life is causing you to feel anxious.
· Take time to dance and sound these sensations.
· Now write quickly: 'I am feeling anxious because…'

- If nothing comes, simply allow the situation to unfold in your life by focusing on the pain or ache and sending light to the pain, ache or sensation.

Exploration: Dancing with Illusion

- Dance with your projections and illusions.
- For stimulus use material that brings up a strong reaction in you, something on screen, on the radio, in a magazine or the newspaper, people in a group you belong to or people you are in relationship with. Take the time to write about this and also be aware of sensations in your body.
- Dance these sensations and take full responsibility for them. These feelings are in your body, they do not belong to the other person. Even if you are picking up energies in other people, it is you who has chosen to tune into these particular energies.
- Afterwards, put paint on paper, let your eyes go into soft focus and look at what you have painted.
- Now write a four-line poem or a song. All energy can be used creatively.

Exploration: Colour and Sound

- Paint using no more than three colours. Put the paint on with your hands or with a brush, you are not trying to make any image but if one comes that is fine.
- When you have finished, close your eyes for a while. See the colours in your mind's eye. Then open your eyes, look at the colours and begin to tone the colour.
- Go close to the colours and then draw away toning and making sound. Sometimes close your eyes and see the colours in your mind's eye and then open them and gaze softly at the colours.
- Afterwards sit in silence for a while.

Exploration: Seeing

· Dance using a veil. Put it in front of your eyes, then slowly take it away.
· Dance putting your hands in front of your eyes and in front of your third eye, also moving your hands in the air around your body and particularly your upper body.
· Let your movements be sacred and bring a quality of stillness to your movements.
· Let your vision open out and slowly let your eyes move from object to object in the room.
· Begin to trace the outline of these objects with your eyes and your hands. Allow your body to follow, breathe.
· Look at the landscape beyond your room and let your eyes trace the tree or the house outside.
· Do this for as long as it feels comfortable. Make sure that you are breathing and that your body is relaxed.
· Look at colours – really see – close your eyes and see that colour in your minds eye.
· Now let your body trace an object, letting your eyes lead. You can make the movements bigger, rising, sinking, curving and shaping your body.
· Gently take your finger and move it upwards on your third eye area as if you were lifting a curtain, and then you can let the curtain fall over this area when you are finished your dance by gently moving your finger downwards.
· If you are dancing with others, you can lift the veil of your own projections on them and ask to see the divine dancer in them. You can also take turns to trace each other's bodies, first of all with your eyes and then with your body. Use different body parts. Remember to breathe.

Exploration: the Shuddering Dance

To release old stuck energy and allow the spirit to enter the body.

· Light your candles, your incense, get your rattles, or whatever is symbolic to you at this time.

- Put on some drumming music and dance through the other colours, all the time observing and scanning the body for pain, numbness, discomfort and the areas of well-being.
- Move with pain, stiffness or coldness in your body, stretch into it and hold it; let your body lead you.
- Follow the shivering or shaking or the rigidity, cold or fear; be gentle.
- Follow the beat of the music, stay down in your hips and legs and dance.
- Shudder and shake until your thoughts are still. You can make ghosty 'hoo hoo' sounds or any sounds that come to you.
- If you are feeling anxious or fearful, you can make quiet time to do this shuddering dance.
- Afterwards, it is important to lie down and rest. Breathe deeply and if you need to, put on some slow safe music. Cover your body with a soft fluffy blanket. Ground your body by feeling your breath pushing your back towards the floor. Hold your hand on your belly and feel it rise and fall with your breath.
- If at any time you feel overwhelmed or nervous, lie on your left side with your knees drawn up. Breathe gently and look around the room, naming the objects you see. Sit up and look outside; name what you see. Go back to base chakra, plant your feet square on the ground, curve over slowly and plant the palms of your hands on the ground. 'I am here now all is well.' Become the animal body, let out a little growl and sink your feet, hands and buttocks into the ground.

Exploration: Respect
- Do you denigrate or jeer at the sacred within? Do you disrespect or make a mockery of it?
- If you receive intuitive messages, do you dismiss them as just imagination?

· Are you afraid of being tricked or conned?
· Can you respect your intuition?
· Were you disciplined as a child? Do you associate discipline with love or lack of love/punishment?
· Do you respect your own soul path and the soul path of others?

Exploration: Protection Cape
· Make a symbolic cape to protect you.
· You can use crêpe paper or material.
· You can stick on symbols or images.
· Wear your cape when you sit down to meditate or hang it on your bedroom door at night.
· Clear and cleanse your cape regularly. You can also use the cape energetically and picture it around your body. Use the colours and symbols that come to you intuitively.
· Make a hood or head covering to protect the antennae around your head.
· Put in a secret opening or aerial that allows you to pick up signals or thoughts that you need to pick up. Use the cape to tune the rest out.
· You can also use light veil-like material to veil your face or any part of your body that feels vulnerable.
· If you work with a lot of people, then afterwards take time to wash your feet and hands in salt water, take a shower and use essential oils – rose, frankincense or lavender – and massage these into your body.
· Clear any old thoughts or anxieties by writing or sharing them with another. Then consciously tune out of the group energy.
· Practise not thinking about people if they are not present. If someone comes into your mind, pause and ask, 'Is there something I need to know?' then either physically contact the person by ringing or writing or tune out the vibration.
· Put a coloured cloth around your phone or your computer

so you are not picking up the calls and emails intuitively unless you need to. When you are ready, then you can check your messages.

· If you have psychic gifts and can see, hear or sense energies, then lower the volume when you are not working so you are not open to energies that do not have your permission to enter. You are also respecting other people's privacy by not tuning into their psyches inappropriately.

Exploration: Resonance

· Are you inclined to resonate with sadness in other people or anger or argumentativeness?
· Notice what emotions you are resonating with in other people. This gives you a clue about how your energy is working and what you are focusing on.
· Notice if you are carrying this energy with you later and own it as your own. Other people are entitled to be sad, tired, etc. without you needing to echo this or to judge.
· Notice in your body where the sensation or feeling is and see if you can let it go by dancing or sounding.

Exploration: the Colour of Dance

· Paint with your fingers to music, let your fingers dance the colours onto the paper.
· Play the same music again and now dance the painting.
· Paint mandalas. Use a plate to draw a circle. Select three colours and paint within the circle. Dance your mandala. Sit in silence and see the mandala in your mind's eye.

Exploration: Ritual Dance

· Create ritual dances to deal with difficulties or losses, or to celebrate your achievements or insights.
· Bring in something that is symbolic to you in your life at

this time; a feather, a stick, a stone. It is very powerful to do this at dusk or into the night.

· Take time to listen to other people's visions. Affirm their dreams.

· Be careful how you use your power. Vows and curses are powerful and can hold us in a bind. Ask to be released from any old vows, e.g. 'I will never love another woman' after your lover has left you. Ritual is very powerful. You can lift these old wishes and curses and also use discernment and wisdom before creating new ones.

· You can also use ritual to protect you from people's bad wishes and thoughts. Songs and dances, for example, the Native American dance 'The Beauty Way' or the old Irish prayer 'The Deers Cry', which has been made into a beautiful song can also protect you. Of course you can also compose your own songs for protection and healing.

· When you are dancing, become conscious of the movements you are making. This heals habitual movement, increases movement memory, and allows new movements to come through.

Exploration: Soul Colours

This exploration is great fun and an easy way to see how intuitive we can be. You can do it on your own, but it is more fun with a group of friends.

· Gather all of your coloured scarves, shawls, wraps, etc. Plain colours are best.

· Choose one person to sit against a neutral background. The person can wear neutral colours but sometimes it is good to see the colours they have chosen already which may not be suiting their aura on that day.

· The rest of the group can stand back and with the eyes in soft focus look at the subject.

· Gently then begin to put a scarf around the person's throat or on their knees. You are looking for the colour that brings the person alive and that warms the skin tone and brings out the eyes.

· This is subtle work. Try different scarves and discard them. Try different combinations, a colour on the legs, around the shoulders, what colour does he/she need around the solar plexus. All the knowledge you have gained while reading this book will rise up. You know this person needs yellow, but today it makes him look sick.

· Find the colours that nurture the person today and that make him/her look at ease, gentled, loved.

· The right colours will light the person up and bring them out of the neutral background.

· You are using colour healing and you are also using all your creativity to find these colours.

· The results are extraordinary. Each person comes into their essence and we can see how beautiful each person can be when they are resonating with their own colours.

· Take turns and work from gentle intuition and try not to get into arguments with each other – it is only a game. Stand back, look, sense, come forward with your colour, then be prepared to see that it might not work. The orange is good but no, it is a little strong. Perhaps you will not have the exact colour, but you can see that if it were a little paler, a peach perhaps and combined with that soft pink on the solar plexus and yes amazingly a touch of turquoise, just there behind the peach and near the eyes. Combine the colours, sometimes a little of this and more of that. Like cooking a dish, a dash of this colour, a pinch of that.

· Sometimes two colours can look great together, for example, a flame red and gold, but you may be combining colours for their own innate beauty and in fact they are not the colours your person needs. Sense the subtle energies; look at the skin and the eyes. Notice if the outline of the body becomes more defined.

· Of course everyone adores this exercise and wants a turn, but don't tire everyone out. You can always do it again.

Exploration: the Five-Minute Healing

This is a simple ritual you can do with a small group of three or more and it follows on beautifully from the previous one.

- One person chooses to lie down and the others choose colours for her/him. Take time to really see and sense the colours this person needs. Try to use scarves that are made from natural material. Cotton, wool, etc. Another person volunteers to do the gypsy reading, while another chooses a divination card for the person receiving the healing.
- Don't be heavy about it, be childlike and simple. This ritual usually only takes five minutes for each person.
- When you have covered the person with the colours, then perhaps add in something significant for the person, e.g. a feather or a stone. Position one person at the feet and another at the head.
- If there are more people you can form a ring around the person. Have your rose oil to hand and you can massage the feet, head and hands.
- Tone into the body for two minutes, looking at the colours as you tone. Allow your voice to move the way it needs to as it will respond intuitively to what the person needs.
- Gently allow the voices to fade away. Have one person leading and watching the time. He or she can give a signal to the group when the time is up.
- Now the gypsy takes her hand and calls for her to come back to the group. The gypsy looks at the palm and speaks for a minute. Letting good wishes and blessings come through in her words.
- Finally, another person chooses a card and shows it to the person receiving the healing. She points out the colours and what the fairies or angels are doing on the card.
- Gently remove the coloured cloths and help the person to get up. Have a blanket ready so he/she can rest and take it all in.
- Now it is someone else's turn.

Exploration: Visualisation

- Scan your body. Notice sensation, stay with it. Let an image come to describe the sensation or emotion, e.g. fear in the third eye – a black key. Strong sensation in the heart – a rainbow going into the earth.
- Start a conversation between the two images. Swap them around. Begin to dance them. Let one lead then the other.
- Let parts of your body speak. Through writing, image, paint, let parts of your body dialogue with other parts.

Exploration: Seeing Blocked Energy in the Body

- Dance through the colours.
- Bounce heels, doing a little trance walk. Keep vision soft, diffuse. Tune into your body and see what part of it your eyes or your inner eye is drawn to.
- Look in the mirror. Your attention may go to some part of your body. Don't criticise. Hold it! This is where the energy is ready to clear. Or you will feel discomfort or pain here. Simply look.
- Same applies when you look at other bodies. Your attention may be drawn to a part of their body. It may be that you are seeing some blocked energy, but draw it back to your own body. If you are looking at the other person's mouth, notice sensation in your own mouth.
- You are looking at bodies as if you are an artist and you could change the shape (energy) with a wave of your brush.

Exploration: Trance Dance

- Do a little trance dance by gently tapping your heels on the ground and making a little sound down low in the body
- Attune with the colour indigo which is the colour of blue ink with purply undertones. Movements are Native American-like. Soft feet.

- Drop the weight downwards, let your body and face be soft, and relaxed. Eyes: soft-focus.
- Make a little repetitive sound, 'Hey Hey-Hey Hey'. Move around the room and let your body be loose, a clackety skeleton bouncing on top of your heels. Your head is loose like a puppet.
- When this feels complete, gather the energy at the top of your head with your arms and hands and put your joined hands on the top of your head, then in front of your forehead, then heart; now gently open your hands and send the energy down into the ground.
- Make a nasal sound in the nose and forehead, like a droning bee sound, or 'nee naw, neeng nong'.

Orange is the complementary colour.

Myth and Ritual

As we dance in the indigo light, each one sees where they have been sabotaging or blocking their vision. We write our stories in myth so that we can come to the truth behind our habitual worries and concerns. We use ritual and mythic language as a way of acknowledging our gifts within the community. In this way, one woman came up with white horses to confront her parents' chaos and fear.

The power of story and myth can be used every day in a simple way with the children and adults around us. We can use myth to make sense of situations we do not understand. When people are called upon to make a myth of their life journeys, they can stumble on truths they were unaware of. One woman was puzzled by a year of her life when she did not have energy to work or even get out of bed. In the myth of her life, she recalled the long journey that had brought her to a small house in the country where she slept and slept and slept. In the myth, the house became a cave and she became a princess who had suffered great trials and who eventually found safety in a cave

– far away and hidden from her tormenters – where she fell into a deep sleep. She slept for four seasons hidden in the dark of the cave and while she slept she had a dream…

The dream in mythical language was the vision for the rest of her life and she could understand it because all the signs and symbols were hers. Myth-making is a tool we use in the third eye and it helps to harmonise the third eye with the throat chakra.

Each person's ritual speaks deeply about his/her journey so far as they gather up their colours and prepare to embark on a new stage of life. Every movement is soft and still, with no unnecessary effort and all is revealed in the turn of a head or eyes looking at you through the dusk or the voices in the trees. This soft veil opens momentarily and you are given a glimpse of bones in a face that is haunted with wisdom, a sound in the undergrowth, the cry of an animal as the moon rises, and everywhere and all around us there are mysterious shapes and shadows, rising and sinking, advancing and retreating.

EXPLORING VIOLET – SACRED DANCE: CHAKRA 7

Key words or clues: crown of head, cerebral cortex, hair, consciousness, pure sensation; movements are sacred mudras and gestures, conscious, still; all movement done with awareness.

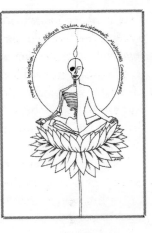

Seventh chakra	crown – thousand-petalled lotus
Element	consciousness
Affirmation	'I Rest in Stillness'
Colours	violet, white, gold, rose and pinky violet, magenta, gold, silver, light and shade
Location	crown – cerebral cortex – hair
Endocrine gland	pineal
Clues	stillness, divine, soul, overview, purification, wisdom, enlightenment, luminous, reverence, inspiration/creativity, mystic, witness, prayer, meditation, attachment/non-attachment, king, queen, goddess, god, compassion, sacrifice, kundalini (the rising serpent of energy that rises up through the chakra system to illumate and enlighten the person) separation, death, shadow, detachment, impersonal love, illumination, acceptance, awe, spiritual power
Discipline	mindfulness
Symbols and props	white candle, tuning fork, sacred book, white lily, lotus, holy grail, eagle, crown, hat, feathers, feathered headdress, sceptre, chalice, violin, gold, amethyst
Fragrance	frankincense, myrrh, lavender

Food	wine, blackberries, grapes, aubergines, purple foods
Imbalances	over-intellectualising, isolating, feeling cut off and separate, disconnected from physical body, mental illness, knowing it all, having all the information, headaches, speedy thoughts, spiritual or religious addiction/abuse, fanaticism, overwhelm, attachment, spiritual cynicism, denial of the shadow, high and mighty, arrogance, inability to ground creative inspiration, misuse of spiritual power

Blackberries that rosaried the hillside,
Untouched by reverent fingers,
purple sluiced their burning bush,
never to stain the pot,
be poured into jam wine.

Eileen Casey

According to ancient esoteric teachings, walking into the violet flame burns away the dross and purifies the whole system. Violet and luminous white light are the spiritual flame. This colour is powerful and often people who are experiencing a spiritual awakening are attracted to the colour violet. We balance the energy with the complementary chakra, the solar plexus, (colour: yellow or gold), and this purifies and balances our body and mind so we can attune with divine inspiration and our soul path. For this reason we use this wavelength sparingly. A little goes a long way. Because of the power of movement, colour and sound, we go very gently in the crown chakra as this fast vibration of light illuminates our shadow.

We may become very still and speaking is an effort. Or we may be in a slightly altered state, there may be a sudden chill of fear, then stillness again. In the crown chakra we are taking an overview – like a great golden eagle soaring above the earth. As we move, we are conscious of the space in and around our

bodies. The movements become very still. Our hands move the
air around our bodies. Our hands might join together in the
prayer position, in front of the heart, in front of the third eye or
over the crown of the head. There is a delicacy in the movement;
a sense of symmetry. As bodies explore the space, it is almost as
if they are being choreographed by a feather-like touch. There
may be strong sensation at the crown of the head, a sense of pure
energy flowing down, through and around the body – like a soft
fresh breeze. Hands move this energy through space and around
the body as we take time to really experience each movement
and the after effects in the body. It is essential to keep the body
grounded so we do not become too floaty. For this reason we
dance for some time through the other colours until we come
to stillness in the crown. We use bells, high music, also music
that resonates through the body, tuning, unifying and balancing.
We are dancing healers. Our hands and bodies move energy as
we touch other bodies and the air around them with reverence.
We are resonating with the energy, like a taut violin string being
plucked by an unseen hand. Sometimes it is almost as if the
body might shatter because the energy coming in is so high and
fine. The mystics speak about the light being so dazzling that
when it was shown to them they begged for it to be taken away.
Sound and light course through the body, throwing shadows
into stark relief, shadows that seem to be polar opposites to
detachment, acceptance and impersonal love. We are conscious
of a loving witness dancing amongst us, willing to ease us of our
burden even though we may be clinging onto it afraid to let go,
afraid to accept that it is time to let go. We must let the flame
burn through the old dross so we can rise free.

We are practising mindfulness in all our movements which
may be sacred, measured, subtle, noble, the wild dance of a gipsy
queen, the ecstatic dance of a dervish or a dancing body twisted
with grief, contracted in fear – light pulsing through human
bone.

In this stillness the way and our destiny is revealed to us. We
may need to shed that which is no longer serving that destiny.

Our energy is balanced, transformed and brought into divine right timing. As we dance through the rainbow colours, we come from this still point and we are lead inexorably towards it.

Music

- The Novus Magnificat, *Through the Stargate*, Constance Demby, Hearts of Space p.o.box 31321, San Francisco, California, 9413
- Sung masses from all cultures
- Gloria, Kyrie, 'Panis Angelicus', Pie Jesu
- Theme music from *The Piano*, Virgin Records. Ltd. Carrington, Composer Michael Nyman, Polydor.
- Gorecki, *Symphony No. 3*,
- Also Aria's from the great operas and classical pieces that resonate with this high vibration, you can research them yourself. Also remember your music from the solar plexus, the hero music from fire dance and the heart music so that you filter down the high tones with balance and compassion.

Working deeply with the violet ray, I have found 'a sensitive pain' – a pain of the soul that is connected to my nervous system. The high sound of violins or the low notes of the cello seem to sing through my body. Inhabiting this high place, I have found the theme music from *Schindler's List*, *Carrington*, or Gorecki's 'Symphony No. 3', seem to resonate with the violet ray, but for balance I might bring in music that resonates with my heart.

Having inhabited these high places, it is essential that we descend back down through the chakras, back down to earth. So bring in the rhythmic grounded music, gospel music or earthy spiritual songs and music.

The Colours Around You – Violet

Violet is the dominant colour in the crown chakra. A person with purple, magenta or violet in their aura shows a highly developed spiritual being. Violet is the colour related to inspiration. Many artists, sensitives and poets are surrounded by this colour when they are receiving higher inspiration. When this inspiration is coming through, you need an outlet however small or you will become sick. Have your colours close to hand, a camera, your pen and notebook or a book of poetry or some inspirational music.

Violet is the ray of purification and sacrifice. Only a few people have this ray in the auric field. Linked to the crown centre and the pineal gland, this ray affects all the chakra centres and the endocrine glands.

The colour violet is good for scalp complaints. It calms and sedates and is good for psychological disturbances and all disorders connected to the nervous system. It also awakens the spiritual and creative impulses. Do not use this ray when you are depressed, instead use pink or green.

In your surroundings violet is good in large rooms or entrance halls, but a little goes a long way. It could be used in curtains or chairs. Use of red and violet is too strong for most people, although as I write I am wearing violet and red; these are often called the Magdalene colours. Red and violet bring the creativity and inspiration through the warm soft earth. You can also use violet and gold or pale violet and green. The colour combination I find particularly healing is pale violet and soft rose pink and I often see these colours when very deep healing work is taking place. Cerise and violet are vibrant and creative. If you are feeling spaced or not really grounded, then you know not to wear this colour. I often see a fine rosy-bluey-pink flooding the room and a pale violet when the atmosphere is filled with impersonal love and very old pain is being healed.

Violet and red make magenta. Magenta and green are considered to be powerful healing colours to use with cancer. They are also good to use after a shock and to polarise the body if the energy has gone too high. Breathe green in horizontally through the heart and magenta through the crown of the head and down to the feet. Use turquoise to calm and sedate.

Exploration: Reclaiming Spiritual Gestures

· Dance now and begin to use spiritual gestures from different traditions.

· Try not to make conditioned or prejudiced responses to the gestures. They are only gestures.

· Instead simply feel what it is like to raise your hands above your head, to give a blessing, to hold your hands open at head level, to form the prayer position, to bow down in abeyance to kneel or to put your head to the floor.

· Slow it all down and simply notice what it is like to occupy this part of the body and the part of the aura around the body. How does it feel to rise, to bow, to hold your hands above your head.

· Raise your hands above your head and draw down the light.

· Often these gestures may rise spontaneously as you dance. However, it is good practice to become mindful and conscious of these movements and their effects on the body without immediately jumping to an interpretation with your thoughts.

· Play sacred music from any tradition or music that is sacred and holy for you. Wait until the movements come. They may be small movements at first. Keep breathing and allow the movement and sound to arise from within.

Exploration: Body Conductor

· Notice the energy moving upwards from the soles of the feet, the feet drawing up the sap and then the energy moving downwards from the crown or getting stuck along the way.

- Where is it stuck? Where do you start thinking? Keep your awareness there.
- Move your hands to that place. Rest there and breathe gently, calming that part of you with a gentle touch.
- What happens if you move your eyes, can you connect that movement of the eyes with your breath?
- What happens if you add conscious movement, or voice?

Exploration: Totem Pole

- Connect with the animal kingdom.
- Meditate on each colour and chakra and ask for your animals to be revealed to you.
- This may not happen straight away and, in fact, it is more powerful if the animals come to you. This may happen in unexpected ways.
- When you have made contact with your animals ask to be shown the teachings of these particular animals in an embodied, sensing way.
- Dance the animals, changing from one to the other. Let these animals relate to each other in your dance.
- Begin with two animals or birds. Let the animals communicate with you and put images on your altar. Allow these animals to communicate to you through your drawings or paintings or through your voice and in your dance.

Exploration: Moving Upwards and Downwards Through the Body Instrument

- You can practise this in your dance – soaring, hovering and then descending.
- See if there is a connection with your sacred gestures.
- Play high music and then low rhythmic music. Notice where it is resonating in your body.
- If you have some time, play the music we suggest for each

chakra from the earth up and make the trip through the colours using only music.

· When you are ready, travel back down using the same music and dancing this time.

· When you are going about your life, take time to pause and be still. What chakra are you playing? What note?

· Which ones are you strong in and where do you need practise?

· Take time to do an inventory. Which chakras are you over-active in, which ones are underactive?

Exploration: Dancing your Dreams

· Record your dreams by writing them in the present tense.

· Notice your body sensations while you were dreaming or as your recall the dream.

· Take time to dance these sensations, even a small gesture or shape, and explore the dream in your body.

· Dance the different characters in your dreams and the interrelationship between them.

· Take time to write or paint afterwards, being conscious all the time of body sensations.

Exploration: Wearing a Crown

· Buy a gold paper crown – the kind used for parties.

· Put it on your head and wear it securely, so you can feel the sensation, especially in the crown of your head.

· Hold a sword or a sceptre. You can make one or simply use a stick/rod. Sense what it is like to have this noble energy flowing from your crown and to be grounded in right action through your sceptre, rod or staff.

· You can point your rod at the earth and feel the energy moving down through you.

· Take time to be a sacred dancer and dance and embody your own light and divinity.

Exploration: Authority and Rebellion
· Find a situation in your life where you are rebelling.
· Dance the authority figure you are rebelling against.
· Now dance the rebel.
· Find a situation in your life where you need to use your authority.
· Dance this authority.
· Now dance the rebel.
· Finally let the two dances come together.
· Look out for situations in your life where you are polarising into one of these. Take time to dance and sound the sensations you associate with these states.
· Explore the ways you rebel, e.g. becoming sleepy, busy, passive, sick, jokey, smart.
· Explore the ways you use your authority, e.g. forcing it on someone else, acting like you know it all, acting superior, reporting them to someone else or talking about their behaviour to someone else.
· Can you use your own inner authority for self-discipline and the ability to act on your own truth and integrity?
· Can you use your rebel to cease behaviour that is no longer helpful to you?

Exploration: Sensitive Touch
· Become still. Breathe easily. Let the tips of your fingers become ultrasensitive. Let your fingers move over your skull, slowly, gently and easily as if you were handling a small animal and checking for injury.
· Feel the pulse at the top of your head and feel this gentle throbbing at your forehead and temples.
· Open and release your jaw, gently moving your fingers around your ears and down the glands on either side of your throat. Finish with one hand on your forehead as if you were checking your temperature and the other hand holding the base of your skull.

- Breathe and hum.
- You can cup the palms of your hands over your eyes too if they feel tight or tense.
- Finally hold your feet in a firm but sensitive way. Sense the energy currents connecting the soles of your feet with the top of your head.
- These instructions are guidelines only. Your own touch will sense out intuitively the points on your skull that need your fingers or the pitch of your humming. Remind yourself to breathe.

Exploration: Shadow Dancing

- Light a candle as it turns dark and begin to dance with the shadows in the room; your own shadow.
- Feel the energy that connects you as you move your arm and the shadow moves its arm.
- Take time to meet and know this shadow.
- If you become too nervous, then gently end the dance and ask your shadow to be patient.
- Otherwise wait until you feel completed. Don't go on for too long – the shadow dance need not be long. Then find an ending. Acknowledge your shadow, give thanks, ask for any messages and make one final shape.
- Afterwards take time to be still.
- Begin to notice shadows, e.g. dappled light dancing on the ground under the trees or the shadows that buildings cast.
- Notice shade and light or the light emanating from the candle and then the darkness around this.
- The shadows under the furniture in your house.
- A face in shadow.
- Explore shadows, dance them, paint them and sing them.
- Get to know the world of shadow and the mirroring shadows everywhere.

Exploration: a Letter From your Shadow

· Having danced with your shadow, take a pen in your non-dominant hand and let your shadow write to you.

· You can also let your shadow paint or draw or work with clay.

· Really go for it, even if your shadow seems shocking to you in some way; hold still and listen.

· If you find this exercise too frightening, then stop but make this a decision. I am stopping now because I choose to. Do not become a victim of it. You can work with your shadow again when you choose to or with support.

· Now write a letter to your shadow.

Exploration: Crown

Take time to reflect on these questions:

· How much of your time is spent in spiritual pursuits?

· Do you have spiritual teachers you look up to and aspire to be like?

· Are you turned off by religion? Are you religious? What do you believe in? Who told you to believe that?

· Do you take time to look at paintings, read or listen to music?

· Do you spend time in nature? Do you feel a connection with the nature around you?

· Are you able to connect with the divine within or are you relying on others to do it for you?

· Are you able to look beyond the everyday world, your family and your immediate concerns and see a bigger picture?

Exploration: Meditation

· Practise this now: close your eyes, look within, what thoughts are dominant, what emotions?

· Are you pulling upwards out of your body?

- Let the energy drop down into the feet, legs and hips.
- Notice the sensations in your body.
- Now sink below that again and notice the tingling.
- You are sinking down into your pure essence, the pure life within your body.
- The heavier sensations will try to pull you away from this essence, or the thoughts and emotions will move and pull you away.
- The more you can stay with this still, pure essence the easier it becomes.
- This essence then moves through the heavier sensations, emotions and thoughts – purifying and clearing.
- This stillness dissolves emotions.
- Perhaps we have been taught that we need to get to the emotion, find where it came from and then get it out of the body.
- Simply touching the emotions and thoughts with this pure, still essence allows that purity to transform the heaviness of the thoughts and emotions and, like homeopathy, bring them back into balance so they resonate with stillness. You may experience this as a light, soft breeze that moves through the denser emotions, giving relief and rest.

Exploration: Grounding Inspiration
Reflect on these questions:

- Do you live in a world of dreams and images and forget about the basics?
- Do you get disoriented and confused or overwhelmed by life?
- Can you become so creative or inspired that you forget to eat, sleep or connect with ordinary life and other people?
- Can you receive inspiration without talking about it, thinking about it or exaggerating it?
- Are you in touch with your inspiration or higher purpose?

- Do you feel disconnected and unable to receive creative ideas or inspiration?
- Do you dismiss other people's creative dreams, visions or experiences as imagination?
- Do you find it hard to listen to people speaking about experiences that do not fall into your experience of every-day life?
- What were your early religious experiences? How did they affect you?
- Were you bullied about religion or told to live to rules that made no sense to you?
- How does this manifest in your life now?
- Do you take time to be still, to reflect, to meditate?

If the creative ideas are no problem but you find it hard to ground them or you become overwhelmed, dance the energy down from the crown and end in an earth dance.

If you are unable to access your creativity, use the higher colours in a small way at first. Have some coloured velvet, felt, or material and touch it every day, move and dance in a sensi-tive, still way. Leave space for doing nothing and connect with nature every day in some small way. Dance upwards from the earth and into the crown.

Exploration: Your Sacred Dance

- Dance through the other chakras and ask for your sacred dance to be revealed to you in the crown chakra. It may come quickly or it may take months to come.
- When it comes, dance it and learn the steps. This is a pow-erful dance for you and you can use it when you need to tune into your soul path or when you need to become still in the midst of pain or confusion.
- Sounds, music or chants may come with the dance. Simply be open to receive the sacred movements and give yourself the time and space to receive them.

Exploration: Attachment

· What are you afraid of losing? Dance your attachment. Now become the object, lifestyle or person you feel attached to and dance that.

· See where the qualities of this person or lifestyle resonate in your own body. Become that. Dance that.

· Go back and dance your longing for this attachment, see where this is in your body.

· Begin a dialogue of movements and sound.

· Now take time to draw back the energy you have given to this attachment. Draw back the qualities to yourself. Does the other person seem to be beautiful, or free or creative?

· Name the qualities now and put a colour to them. Now ask for these qualities to come fully alive within you.

· Notice energy lines connecting you to the object of your attachment. If you feel ready, begin to dissolve these energy lines as you dance.

Exploration: Soul Voice

· When you are resonating with the violet flame and the experience of transcendence, tone through the chakras, letting the sounds come without censorship.

· Let your mouth move and feel your voice in different parts of your body.

· Breathe in all the colours and then the colour gold and see this colour cascading down through and around your body.

· Let words and sounds come; do not censor them. Listen.

Exploration: Dancing for Others

· If there is someone you wish to dance for, simply picture them in your mind or use a photograph.

· Focus on the person. You are not trying to change them or affect them in any way, your dance is a gift.

- Allow your body to move gently and trust the movements that come.
- When the dance feels complete, find an ending for your dance and let a name for it bubble up from inside.
- You could then make a card or a small clay figure, a doll or a painting or poem, and send it to the person with a record of your dance. 'I danced for you on Monday the 18th at 2.00 p.m. I offer this dance to you as a gift.'
- If there is a situation that concerns you, then dance for that situation: perhaps a child who is hungry or sick, or a family you know who are affected by addiction or past trauma, or an environmental concern.
- You can add chanting and singing to that, and you could also organise a group of people to dance and sing for that situation. All of you dancing with good intention will create a circle of peace.
- Do not decide with your thoughts what the outcome should be; simply accept the situation, surrender and let the dance be an empathetic and artistic expression of your relationship with these people and their situation.

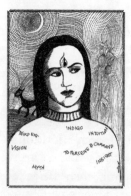

Conclusion

There is an old Buddhist saying 'After the ecstasy, the laundry'. To be able to be present to the daily earthy tasks and to bring a presence and stillness to the washing, the gardening or minding the children, this to me is a sweet thing because I was often in so much emotional pain I could not be present to these tasks. To be able to use all that we have learned while we dance; that is our task. To be conscious in the body as you sweep the floor, or hang clothes on the line, drive the car or type on the computer – all of this is a beautiful dance.

After the high tones of the crown, we need to do the laundry. While we do it, we can put on our music, have the book near and practise a few little movements or sounds. The writing in the section, 'Dancing with the Instinctual Body' has focused on the first chakra as a way of grounding the body and it is good practice to come home to that ground again having explored any of the other colours. If you need balance and ease, dance the gentle movements in the heart or simply play some heart music as you go about your day. Some gentle lullabies can help us to come home to the heart and be comforted if we are feeling afraid. If you need to speak up for yourself then go to the blue section and practice your favourite explorations. If you need to work on your relationships then the orange, fluid dance will help you with this.

When I was a child, we used to gather all the children in

246

our housing estate together and we would sing and dance. Our stage was a giant piece of old board and we used to make our parents bring their own chair and pay to see these concerts on the grass. We took ourselves and our playing very seriously. The cast were aged two to twelve. In each face there was boldness, fun, curiosity, sadness and the fear of being left out. There were bossy ones, quiet ones and ones that caused trouble. I assumed they could all sing and dance and make costumes and create, so they did. We all got paid out of the takings. We had a place to live, a hut in the trees and we bought cake to eat and books for our library.

Over the years it seems to me that the child within us is often the one who holds the keys to why we do the things we do. She is also the one who can see though the bullshit and she knows if I am being authentic or not. When we play, we reach the magical child within and also the child who is confused and hurt. When we go back and play, we find ways to heal and change. Life becomes simpler and easier. It does not matter if your playing is something they rave about in the newspapers or if it happens in private with your colours and your scarves.

When Antoinette and I met over our first cup of tea, the conversation turned easily and naturally to the way we were as children. I remember Antoinette saying that as a child she felt she must be here to do something really important because she was born on 21 June, the longest day, and her name was so long. She recalled how once, when she was sitting on the back step beside the milk bottles, she looked around the garden and felt … something. Confidences flew out of our mouths. A stillness came over us, an echo of the children we once were and the bodies we had then. Antoinette began to work with rhythm by shaking a matchbox and dancing round the room and that led to drumming in Ireland and Africa and seeing the dance dream being lived every day. I began a warrior dance, brandishing my spear, the sweeping brush, and that led to me dancing in the sun palace in Mexico with the Aztec warriors and being able to use the sword of my pen to cut through the undergrowth.

Whenever I hear people speaking about the way they were as children, a world of wonder opens up for me as I see the natural wisdom and creativity I had in the midst of games and dreams. And so it begins and ends with playing; playing with dreams and grounding the dreaming in the dance. This dance is truly an alchemical journey through the senses and the rainbow body; may it be as magical and playful for you as it has been for me.

As the music fades then, we can find a good finish for our dance, a hand raised, a foot poised, the turn of a head, a drum roll, a flash of colour, the click of a castanet, and it is over. As the curtain falls, the only applause that really matters is our own and the knowledge that we really did dance our dreams.

Further Reading

Cameron, Julia, *Walking in this World* (Tarcher/Putnam, 2002)

Anodea, Judith, *Eastern Body – Western Mind* (Celestial Arts Publishing, 1996)

Levine, Peter A. and Fredrick, Ann, *Waking the Tiger – Healing Trauma* (North Atlantic Books, 1997)

Laban, Rudolf, *The Language of Movement* (Boston Plays Inc, 1974)

Khan, Hazrat Inayat, *The Mysticism of Sound and Music* (Servire BV, 1979)

Feldenkrais, Moshe, *Awareness through Movement* (Harper Collins, 1972–1990)

Brennan, Richard, *The Alexander Technique Manual* (Eddison Sadd Editions, 1996)

Caldwell, Christine, *Getting our Bodies Back* (Shambala Publications, 1996)

Payne, Helen, *Creative Movement and Dance in Groupwork* (Winslow Press, 1990)

Corry, Dr. Michael, Tubridy, Dr. Aine, *Depression, An Emotion not a Disease.* (Mercier Press, 2005)

Wright, Machaelle Small, *Behaving As If the God in All Life Mattered* (Jeffersonton, Va, Perelandra Ltd, 1987)

McLeod, June, *Colours of the Soul* (Piatkus, 2000)

Hart, Mickey, *Drumming at the Edge of Magic* (Harper Collins, 1990)

Roth, Gabrielle and Loudon, John, *Maps to Ecstasy Teachings of an Urban Shaman* (Novato, Calif, Nataraj Publishing, 1989)

Bibliography

Rumi, Rabindranath and Tagore, Wovoka 'The Ghost Dance' taken from *Poetry Quotes*

Thomson, Belinda. (editor) *Gauguin by himself*, (Time Warner Books, 2004)

Khan, Hazrat Inayat. *The Mysticism of Sound and Music*, (Servire BV, 1979)

Levine, Peter A. and Frederick, Ann. *Waking the Tiger: Healing Trauma*, (North Atlantic Books, 1997)

Page, Dr. Christine. *Frontiers of Health*, (C.W. Daniel Company Ltd, 1992)

Fennell, Jan. *The Practical Dog Listener*, (Harper Collins, 2002)

Anodea, Judith. *Eastern Body Western Mind-Psychology and the Chakra System*, (Celestial Arts Publishing, 1996)

Caldwell, Christine. *Getting our Bodies Back*, (Shambala publications, 1996)

Jodjana, Raden Ayou. *A Book of Self Re-Education, The Structure and Functions of the Human Body as an Instrument of Expression*, , L.N., (Fowler & Co. Ltd.)

Keenan, Brian. *An Evil Cradling*, (Penguin, 1994)

Harris, Joanne. *Chocolat*, (Black Swan, 2000)

Diamant, Anita. *The Red Tent*, (Pam Books, 2002)

Bly, Robert, *News of the Universe* (Sierra Club Books, 1980)

Acknowledgements

For initial editorial input and advice I would like to thank Colin Morrison, Liz Puttick, Gill Farrer Halls, Jill Riordan and Sara Smith. I would also like to thank Mary Feehan for believing in miracles and the integrity and experience she brought to editing what was initially a huge tome. My heartfelt thanks to her and all the team at Mercier Press for making me so welcome and giving me such professional help. Thank you also to John, my love, for putting up with and nurturing me through all the years it took to get this knowledge down on paper and to Michelle, Louise, Emer and Elaine, for your belief in me.

Dancing the Rainbow course – Acknowledgements

Dancing the Rainbow courses, workshops and trainings were designed and developed by Antoinette Spillane and I. Some of the explorations I use come from those we have used in our joint work and often our voices harmonise together. For the sake of fluidity I have not tried to isolate her input, indeed at this stage that would be difficult. Antoinette's vision comes right through the work. I would also like to thank John Doyle who was and is Vision maker and guide. Deirdre O'Connor and Joanne Ni Bhaoill who are now communing deeply with the work and adding new insights; also Dara Skuse, Maura Horkan, Patricia Nugent, Mary Lys Carberry, Torsten Eisenberg and Majella Canning. And thank you to all the beautiful Rainbow dancers and teachers, each and everyone, your courage, creativity, personal research and input has been invaluable. I would also like to thank the people who have supported us with delicious wholefood and/or beautiful surroundings as we danced.

Lastly I acknowledge and thank those teachers, dancers, mentors, family and friends who have contributed their knowledge, skill and support to my life and work: in particular members of the St. Colmcilles Writers Group, Marie Louise Lacey, Mary Stewart, Mo Griffiths, Joan Davis, Ray Smith and most especially Patricia Quinn for the healing of this body and Derry McDermot for her wisdom, skill, love and compassion over many years as I worked with and healed my own roots.

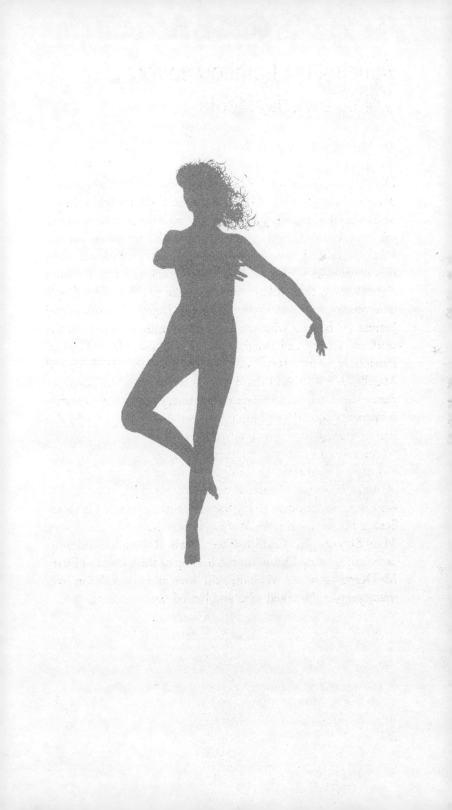

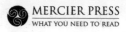
Depression
An Emotion not a Disease

Dr Michael Corry
Dr Áine Tubridy

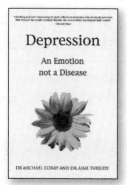

ISBN: 978 1 85635 479 0

Is there any end to the cycle of relapse, hospitalisation and medication for sufferers of depression? Drs Michael Corry and Áine Tubridy believe there is.

In this hard-hitting book, Corry and Tubridy present a revolutionary new perspective in which they assert that depression is an emotion, just like fear, anger or love, that can be consciously influenced, rather than a disease which can only be suffered.

This new theory has enormous implications for the traditional treatment of depression. It puts the sufferer back at the centre of a more individual and tailored approach to healing and raises serious questions about the medical community's focus on medication as a primary treatment.

Depression speaks both to those experiencing depression and to their families. Its aim is to:
*   offer hope and understanding;
*   equip sufferers with the resources to buffer them against future setbacks;
*   end the cycle of relapse and remediate;
*   provide effective ways to create a new identity for the sufferer, rooted in self-acceptance and empowerment.

Michael Corry, MD, a psychiatrist, and Áine Tubridy, MD, a psychotherapist, are practising and living in Ireland. Their previous books are *Going Mad?* and *When Panic Attacks*.

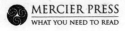

When Heaven Answers
Stories of Hope and Healing

Teresa Nerney
Foreword by Heather Parsons

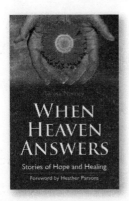

ISBN: **978 1 85635 532 2**

When nobody on earth could help … heaven answered their prayers

In *When Heaven Answers* Irish people, young and old, share remarkable and inspirational stories of faith, hope and healing.

They are heart-wrenching stories: Alice Cairns describes how she was healed after experiencing a mother's worst nightmare, when her teenage son went missing without trace. Marion Carroll was on death's door when she arrived at Knock Shrine in 1989. Here she reflects on her miraculous recovery from multiple sclerosis. Michael Woods desperately wished for a cure for his wife Rita's alzheimers, until healing came in a most unexpected way.

Teresa Nerney reveals how heaven answered their prayers, and the prayers of many others, in this poignant collection of interviews and stories from inspirational people who have conquered unimaginable challenges and sadness in their lives.

When Heaven Answers reminds us that we are never alone, and never without hope, no matter how painful and difficult our circumstances may be.

Teresa Nerney is a journalist and author living in the west of Ireland. She writes weekly for the RTÉ Guide magazine and contributes to and edits a number of publications.

Heather Parsons, who is recognised as one of the best-known commentators on the apparitions at Medjugorje, writes the Foreword.